T0263123

Correction of Multiplanar Deformity of the Foot and Ankle

Guest Editor

ANISH R. KADAKIA, MD

FOOT AND ANKLE CLINICS

www.foot.theclinics.com

Consulting Editor

MARK S. MYERSON, MD

September 2009 • Volume 14 • Number 3

SAUNDERS an imprint of ELSEVIER, Inc.

W.B. SAUNDERS COMPANY
A Division of Elsevier Inc.

1600 John F. Kennedy Blvd. • Suite 1800 • Philadelphia, PA 19103-2899

http://www.theclinics.com

FOOT AND ANKLE CLINICS Volume 14, Number 3
September 2009 ISSN 1083-7515, ISBN-10: 1-4377-1217-7, ISBN-13: 978-1-4377-1217-9

Editor: Debora Dellapena

Foot and Ankle Clinics (ISSN 1083-7515) is published quarterly by Elsevier, Inc., 360 Park Avenue South, New York, NY 10010-1710. Months of issue are March, June, September, and December. Customer Service Office: Health Sciences Division, Subscription Customer Service, 3251 Riverport Lane, Maryland Heights, MO 63043. Periodicals postage paid at New York, NY, and additional mailing offices. Subscription price per year is $230.00 (US individuals), $333.00 (US institutions), $116.00 (US students), $257.00 (Canadian individuals), $394.00 (Canadian institutions), $159.00 (Canadian students), $331.00 (foreign individuals), $394.00 (foreign institutions), and $159.00 (foreign students). To receive student/resident rate, orders must be accompanied by name of affiliated institution, date of term, and the *signature* of program/residency coordinator on institution letterhead. Orders will be billed at individual rate until proof of status is received. Foreign air speed delivery is included in all *Clinics* subscription prices. All prices are subject to change without notice. **POSTMASTER:** Send address changes to *Foot and Ankle Clinics*, Elsevier Health Sciences Division, Subscription Customer Service, 3251 Riverport Lane, Maryland Heights, MO 63043. **Customer Service: 1-800-654-2452 (US and Canada). From outside of the United States and Canada, call 314-447-8871. Fax: 314-417-8029. E-mail: Journals CustomerService-usa@elsevier.com (for print support); JournalsOnlineSupport-usa@elsevier.com (for online support).**

Reprints. For copies of 100 or more, of articles in this publication, please contact the Commercial Reprints Department, Elsevier Inc., 360 Park Avenue South, New York, NY 10010-1710. Tel.: 212-633-3812; Fax: 212-462-1935; E-mail: reprints@elsevier.com.

Printed and bound in the United Kingdom
Transferred to Digital Print 2011

Contributors

CONSULTING EDITOR

MARK S. MYERSON, MD
Director, The Institute for Foot and Ankle Reconstruction, Mercy Medical Center, Baltimore, Maryland

GUEST EDITOR

ANISH R. KADAKIA, MD
Chief, Department of Orthopaedic Surgery, Division of Foot and Ankle Surgery; Assistant Professor, University of Michigan, Ann Arbor, Michigan

AUTHORS

ADAM S. BECKER, MD
Director, Institute for Foot and Ankle Reconstruction, Mercy Medical Center, Baltimore, Maryland; Englewood Orthopaedic Associates, Englewood, New Jersey

MARCO TÚLIO COSTA, MD
Instructor, Professor, and Attending Physician, Department of Orthopaedics, Division of Foot and Ankle, Santa Casa School of Medicine and Hospitals, São Paulo, Brazil.

MICHAEL J. COUGHLIN, MD
Director, Idaho Foot and Ankle Fellowship; Clinical Professor, Oregon Health Sciences University, Boise, Idaho

BRYAN D. DEN HARTOG, MD
Assistant Clinical Professor, Sanford School of Medicine; Black Hills Orthopaedic and Spine Center, Rapid City, South Dakota

THOMAS DREHER, MD
Department of Orthopaedics, Division of Pediatric Orthopaedics and Foot Surgery, University of Heidelberg, Heidelberg, Germany

RICARDO CARDENUTO FERREIRA, MD
Director, Division of Foot and Ankle, Santa Casa School of Medicine and Hospitals; Assistant Professor, Department of Orthopaedics, Santa Casa School of Medicine and Hospitals, São Paulo, Brazil.

SEBASTIÉN HAGMANN, MD
Department of Orthopaedics, Division of Pediatric Orthopaedics and Foot Surgery, University of Heidelberg, Heidelberg, Germany

DAVID B. KAY, MD
Associate Professor of Orthopaedic Surgery, Northeast Ohio University College of Medicine, Rootstown, Ohio

ANDRES KELLER, MD
Department of Foot and Ankle Surgery, Clinica Alemana and Padre Hurtado Hospital;
Associate Professor, Universidad del Desarrollo, Santiago, Chile

METIN KUCUKKAYA, MD
Associate Professor, Department of Orthopaedics and Traumatology, Sisli Etfal Research
and Training Hospital, Istanbul, Turkey

UNAL KUZGUN, MD
Professor and Chief, Department of Orthopaedics and Traumatology, Sisli Etfal Research
and Training Hospital, Sisli, Istanbul, Turkey

ANDREW PETER MOLLOY, MR, FRCS (Tr & Orth)
University Hospital Aintree, Lower Lane, Liverpool, United Kingdom

MARK S. MYERSON, MD
Director, Attending Orthopaedic Surgeon, The Institute for Foot and Ankle
Reconstruction, Mercy Medical Center, Baltimore, Maryland

BADRI NARAYAN, MR, FRCS (Tr & Orth)
Consultant Orthopaedic Surgeon, Royal Liverpool University Hospital, Liverpool, United
Kingdom

CRISTIAN ORTIZ, MD
Chief of Foot and Ankle Surgery, Clinica Alemana; Associate Professor, Universidad del
Desarrollo, Santiago, Chile

GEORGE E. QUILL, Jr., MD
Director of Foot and Ankle Services, Louisville Orthopaedic Clinic; Assistant Clinical
Professor of Orthopaedic Surgery, Department of Orthopaedic Surgery, University
of Louisville School of Medicine, Louisville, Kentucky

ANDY ROCHE, MR, MRCS
Specialist Registrar in Orthopaedics, University Hospital Aintree, Lower Lane, Liverpool,
United Kingdom

V. JAMES SAMMARCO, MD
Cincinnati Sports Medicine and Orthopaedic Center, Cincinnati, Ohio

BERTIL W. SMITH, MD
Assistant Clinical Professor, Chief, Foot and Ankle Surgery Program, Department
of Orthopaedic Surgery, University of California San Diego, San Diego, California

EMILIO WAGNER, MD
Department of Foot and Ankle Surgery, Clinica Alemana and Padre Hurtado Hospital;
Associate Professor, Universidad del Desarrollo, Santiago, Chile

WOLFRAM WENZ, MD
Head, Department of Orthopaedic Surgery, Division of Pediatric Orthopaedics and Foot
Surgery, University of Heidelberg, Heidelberg, Germany

Contents

Treatment of Hallux Valgus with Increased Distal Metatarsal Articular Angle: Use of Double and Triple Osteotomies

Bertil W. Smith and Michael J. Coughlin

The treatment of the congruent hallux valgus deformity requires special consideration for a successful outcome to be obtained. The distal metatarsal articular angle is of critical importance in this deformity. The goal of correction is to achieve a realigned first ray and preserve the congruent first metatarsophalangeal articulation. In patients with an increased distal metatarsal articular angle and congruent joint, the use of double and triple first ray osteotomies must be used to achieve satisfactory correction.

Non-Neuropathic Midfoot Multiplanar Deformity: Surgical Strategies for Reconstruction

Bryan D. Den Hartog and David B. Kay

The most common multiplanar deformity of the midfoot is pes planovalgus. Clinically, the flatfoot is characterized by a depressed or absent medial longitudinal arch accompanied by forefoot abduction and, in some cases, by supination of the forefoot and valgus angulation of the hindfoot. This article reviews the reconstructive strategies for correction of deformity and fusion of the painful arthritic joints. A stepwise surgical approach is recommended for reproducible correction and midfoot fusion in patients with arthritis combined with a multiplanar deformity. The article focuses on the principles of reconstruction of the planovalgus deformity in the non-neuropathic patient using compression plates for a stable construct fixation.

Superconstructs in the Treatment of Charcot Foot Deformity: Plantar Plating, Locked Plating, and Axial Screw Fixation

V. James Sammarco

Management of Charcot's deformity of the foot and ankle continues to challenge physicians. Medical co-morbidity, peripheral neuropathy, vascular disease, and immune impairment cause severe problems for these patients and, when combined with neuroarthropathy, can lead to amputation. Progressive bony deformity and bone resorption, which may accompany neuroarthropathy, only increase the challenge of surgical treatment. These challenges have led physicians to develop "superconstruct" techniques to improve fixation, whereby fusion is extended beyond the zone of injury to include joints that are not affected, bone resection is performed to shorten the extremity to allow for adequate reduction of deformity without undue tension on the soft tissue envelope, the strongest device is used that can be tolerated by the soft tissue envelope; and the devices are applied in a novel position that maximizes mechanical function. This article reviews three techniques designed to achieve lasting deformity correction and successful arthrodesis: plantar plating, locked plating, and axial screw fixation.

Skewfoot is a rare deformity characterized by forefoot adduction and hindfoot valgus. Its etiology and natural history are unknown, although congenital and syndromic forms are observed. Currently, there is no consent about the treatment of skewfoot. Due to its potential resistance to the effects of therapy, it must be differentiated from other, more common deformities. Treatment involves conservative and, most often, operative measures.

A simplified standard setting of the circular external fixator allows correction of all the complex deformities of recurrent clubfoot with minimal surgical intervention and no major complications. In those cases where additional corrective arthrodesis is necessary, it is performed with minimal bone resection because the severe deformities of the foot and ankle have already been corrected.

A multiplanar foot deformity is defined by the presence of more than one deformity affecting the foot. These deformities may develop in any plane, including the frontal, sagittal, or transverse planes. This article focuses on the treatment of multiplanar neuromuscular foot deformities with external fixation, reviewing the indications, preoperative planning, techniques, and complications.

This article presents a surgical protocol for surgical reconstruction from the subtle cavus foot described by Manoli to the most complicated cases. The goal is to merge together the available surgical options in a comprehensive way to guide surgical decisions.

Reconstruction surgery of the midand hindfoot is a demanding challenge for foot surgeons. Satisfactory results depend not only on surgical technique and skills but also on the knowledge of underlying disorders, pathomechanics, and indication criteria. The cavovarus foot, the planovalgus foot, and Charcot's foot are some of the most challenging foot deformities, requiring different surgical strategies for their correction. Most of the osteotomies and fusions in children and adults can be fixed with transcutaneous Kirschner wires, which are inexpensive and easy to use and remove. The use of alternative fixation systems such as cannulated screws, compression screws, or angle-stable locking plates depends on patient age, vascular situation, risk for nonunion, and underlying pathology.

THE CLINICS ARE NOW AVAILABLE ONLINE!

Access your subscription at:
www.theclinics.com

Preface

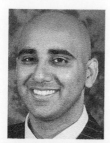

Anish R. Kadakia, MD
Guest Editor

Deformity correction is a complex and rewarding surgical challenge. Multiplanar deformities are particularly difficult, requiring an in-depth understanding not only of the radiographic abnormalities but also of the underlying pathogenesis. Surgical correction must address each component in the ankle, hindfoot, midfoot, and forefoot to create a functional limb. The presence of multiple sites of deformity requires thorough preoperative planning and a systematic approach to be successful. The contribution of muscular imbalance, ligamentous instability, bony abnormality, presence of degenerative changes, and prior surgery must be taken into account. The method of fixation must be considered, as this may determine the type of osteotomy that is required.

The complex and uncommon nature of these conditions makes it difficult for a single surgeon to become adept in dealing with the multitude of pathologies. The authors in this issue of *Foot and Ankle Clinics of North America* are experts in dealing with multiplanar deformities, each one specializing in a unique condition and fixation technique. By sharing the knowledge and experience of our colleagues, each of us can expand our ability to treat these complex deformities. I would like to commend the authors on the tremendous time and effort that they put forth in preparation of their articles. I would also like to thank Dr. Myerson and everyone at Elsevier for their help in putting this issue together. I sincerely hope that you enjoy this issue and that the authors' efforts assist in the treatment of your patients.

Anish R. Kadakia, MD
Chief
Department of Orthopedic Surgery
Division of Foot and Ankle Surgery
Assistant Professor
University of Michigan
2098 South Main Street
Ann Arbor, MI 48103, USA

E-mail address:
anishk@med.umich.edu (A.R. Kadakia)

Foot Ankle Clin N Am 14 (2009) ix
doi:10.1016/j.fcl.2009.07.001
1083-7515/09/$ – see front matter

Treatment of Hallux Valgus with Increased Distal Metatarsal Articular Angle: Use of Double and Triple Osteotomies

Bertil W. Smith, MD[a,b,]*, Michael J. Coughlin, MD[c,d]

KEYWORDS

• Hallux valgus • Congruent • Juvenile • Articular • Deformity

Carl Heuter first coined the term "hallux valgus" in 1871.[1] He defined it as a subluxation of the first metatarsophalangeal (MTP) joint with lateral deviation of the great toe and medial deviation of the first metatarsal. It is the most common problem affecting the great toe. As many as 2% to 4% of the population are affected with the deformity,[2] and more than 90% of the patients are women.[3–6]

The cause of the hallux valgus deformity is multifactorial and, with rare exception, it occurs in shoe-wearing cultures.[7–12] One study from China reported a 15-fold higher incidence of hallux valgus in persons who wore shoes compared with persons who did not.[13] Another study from Japan noted a significant increase in the hallux valgus deformity after the introduction of high fashion footwear after World War II.[14] Genetics also plays a major role, with a positive family history being reported in many series.[3–6,15–28] Coughlin and Jones[3] recently reported on the demographics and natural history of hallux valgus. They noted that 84% of patients had a positive family history, most commonly from maternal transmission, with 27% of patients reporting a three-generation history of the deformity. Hardy and Clapham[6] similarly reported that 77% of patients in their series noted that their mother had bunions.

---

[a] Foot and Ankle Surgery Program, Department of Orthopaedic Surgery, University of California, San Diego, 350 Dickinson Street, Suite 121, San Diego, CA 92103-8894, USA
[b] Department of Orthopaedic Surgery, University of California, San Diego, 200 W. Arbor Dr., MC#8894, San Diego, CA 92103-8894, USA
[c] Idaho Foot and Ankle Fellowship, 901 N. Curtis Road, Suite 503, Boise, ID 83706, USA
[d] Oregon Health Sciences University, 901 N. Curtis Road, Suite 503, Boise, ID 83706, USA
* Corresponding author. Department of Orthopaedic Surgery, University of California, San Diego, 200 W. Arbor Dr., MC#8894, San Diego, CA 92103-8894.
E-mail address: batsmithmd@hotmail.com (B.W. Smith).

Foot Ankle Clin N Am 14 (2009) 369–382
doi:10.1016/j.fcl.2009.03.005
1083-7515/09/$ – see front matter © 2009 Elsevier Inc. All rights reserved.

foot.theclinics.com

The classification of hallux valgus depends on several patient factors and angular measurements, including the hallux valgus angle, 1-2 intermetatarsal (IM) angle, hallux valgus interphalageus angle, and distal metatarsal articular angle (DMAA) **(Fig. 1A–C)**.[29] Using these angular measurements, the deformity is classified as mild, moderate, or severe. A mild deformity is defined as a hallux valgus angle less than 20° and 1-2 IM angle less than or equal to 11°. With a moderate deformity, the hallux

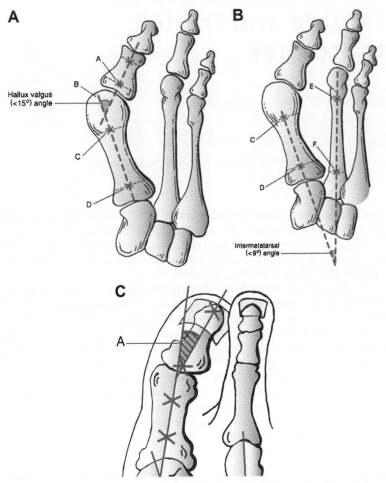

Fig.1. (A) Hallux valgus angle. Marks are placed in the mid-diaphyseal region of the proximal phalanx and the first metatarsal at an equal distance from the medial and lateral cortices. The hallux valgus angle is formed by the intersection of the diaphyseal axes of the first metatarsal (line CD) and the proximal phalanx (line AB). (B) 1-2 IM angle. Mid-diaphyseal reference points are placed equidistant from the medial and lateral cortices of the first and second metatarsals in the proximal and distal mid-diaphyseal regions. The 1-2 IM angle is formed by the intersection of these two axes (line CD and line EF). (C) Hallux valgus interhpalangeus angle. Mid-diaphyseal reference points are drawn on the proximal and distal phalanx. The intersection of the axis of the distal phalanx with the longitudinal axis of the proximal phalanx forms the hallux valgus interphalangeus angle. (*From* Coughlin MJ. Hallux valgus. In: Coughlin MJ, Mann RA, Saltzman CL, editors. Surgery of the foot and ankle. 8th edition. Philadelphia: Mosby-Elsevier; 2007. p. 209; with permission.)

valgus angle ranges between 20° and 40° with the 1-2 IM angle being less than 16°. A severe deformity is defined as a hallux valgus angle more than 40° with the 1-2 IM angle being more than 16°. The DMAA allows the deformity to be classified as subluxated or congruent, with a DMAA of less than 6° defined as normal.[30,31]

Although most hallux valgus deformities result from progressive subluxation of the first MTP joint, deformity also may result from a sloped angle of the distal metatarsal articular surface resulting in an increased distal metatarsal articular angle. The DMAA is measured on the anteroposterior radiograph. To measure the DMAA, a line is drawn from the most medial extent of the metatarsal articular surface to its most lateral extent. This line defines the lateral slope of the articular surface. A perpendicular line is then drawn to this articular line. The angle between this perpendicular line and the long axis of the metatarsal is known as the DMAA (**Fig. 2**). The congruency of the joint is determined by evaluating the relationship of the metatarsal head articular surface to the articular surface of the base of the proximal phalanx. With a subluxated deformity, the articular surface of the base of the proximal phalanx is deviated laterally from the metatarsal articular surface. With a congruent deformity, the articular surfaces match. In this case, the magnitude of the hallux valgus deformity matches that of the DMAA.

Although the interobserver reliability is high with respect to the hallux valgus angle and 1-2 IM angle,[32,33] the same cannot be said about the DMAA.[32,34] Chi and colleagues[35] also found difficulty in the accuracy of assessing joint congruency. Richardson and colleagues[36] were able to reliably quantify the DMAA radiographically.

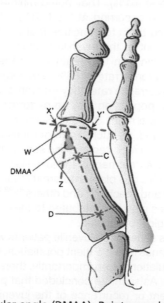

Fig. 2. Distal metatarsal articular angle (DMAA). Points are placed on the most medial and lateral extent of the distal metatarsal articular surface (X',Y'). Another line through points (W, Z) is drawn perpendicular to the first line X'- Y'. A third line through points (C, D) defines the longitudinal axis of the first metatarsal. The angle subtended by the perpendicular line (W, Z), and longitudinal axis of the first metatarsal (C, D) defines the DMAA. (*From* Coughlin MJ. Hallux valgus. In: Coughlin MJ, Mann RA, Saltzman CL, editors. Surgery of the foot and ankle. 8th edition. Philadelphia: Mosby-Elsevier; 2007. p. 210; with permission.)

Joint congruency is more difficult to evaluate radiographically in skeletally immature patients, however.

Piggot[37] was the first to recognize the difference between a congruent and subluxated first MTP joint. He noted that the articular surfaces of the base of the proximal phalanx and metatarsal head are not truly at 90° in relation to the diaphysis, which results in the valgus angle seen in a normal foot without subluxation. He noted that with a congruent hallux valgus deformity, the entire valgus angle is the result of a tilting of the articular surface. He reported an incidence of a congruent joint in 9% of cases in his series. He did not, however, define or measure the DMAA. He concluded that a congruent deformity was more stable and that the hallux valgus was less likely to increase with time. Coughlin[3] also reported a 7% incidence of a congruent joint in his series of patients with hallux valgus.

The association between constricting shoe wear and the hallux valgus deformity does not seem as strong in the juvenile population.[6,38,39] Coughlin[16] noted that 24% of juvenile hallux valgus patients implicated constricting footwear as contributing to the deformity. The age of onset of the deformity is a significant predictor of the congruency of the joint and magnitude of the DMAA. Patients with an onset of deformity before 10 years old had a significantly increased magnitude of hallux valgus deformity and DMAA.

The treatment of a congruent hallux valgus deformity has not been without controversy. The failure rate of surgical intervention of juvenile hallux valgus deformity is reported to be high.[4,18,21,23,28,40,41] Ball and Sullivan[40] reported on the use of the Mitchell osteotomy for correction of the juvenile bunion deformity. In their series of 12 patients treated with a total of 18 osteotomies, a recurrence of the hallux valgus deformity was noted in 11 feet (61%). They noted maintenance of correction of the 1-2 IM angle, with recurrence occurring at the MTP joint with an increasing hallux valgus angle. Their results led them to conclude that the Mitchell osteotomy should be abandoned in the treatment of the juvenile bunion. Scranton and Zuckerman[28] also reported on their experience in the treatment of the adolescent hallux valgus deformity. They noted a recurrence rate of 36% with surgical correction of 50 feet in 31 patients. With this high recurrence rate, they recommended that surgical treatment of bunions in the adolescent population only be performed in the setting of progressive, painful deformity. At the time of Ball and Scranton's early reports, the DMAA had not yet been described and, as such, was not measured and reported.

With the high recurrence rates reported in these series, there has been considerable reservation about the operative treatment of the juvenile bunion deformity. Some have suggested an association with a pes planus deformity that contributes to the development of hallux valgus. Kalen and Brecher[42] and others[20,23,24,27,28,42–46] concluded that an increased incidence of pes planus contributed to the occurrence and risk of recurrence of deformity after surgical correction.

Coughlin[16] reported on his series of 45 juvenile patients with hallux valgus and noted a 17% occurrence of pes planus in this patient population, which was no different than that seen in the normal population. More importantly, there was no recurrence seen in the presence of pes planus. As such, he concluded that pes planus played no significant role in the development or recurrence of the juvenile hallux valgus deformity. A similar conclusion was reached in his reports on adult hallux valgus deformities in which he noted an incidence of pes planus in 15% of patients.[3,47] Kilmartin and Wallace[48] also examined the effect of pes planus and its role in the development of hallux valgus in children. They evaluated a group of 32 11-year-old children with hallux valgus compared with a group of 11-year-old children without first MTP joint deformity. No association could be found linking pes planus to the hallux valgus deformity.

The surgical treatment of juvenile bunion deformities dates back more than 100 years. Kelikian[1] lists more than 100 operations for the treatment of adolescent hallux valgus. Carr and colleagues[49] reported on their use of the Mitchell osteotomy with 54 adolescent feet included in the cohort. The youngest patient to undergo surgical correction in this group was 10 years old. At final follow-up (2–8 years) they rated 41 feet as having excellent results. Looking more carefully at the data collected, there is no mention of the hallux valgus angle in these patients. The cause of the deformity was thought to be from metatarsus primus varus, and as such, the correction of the 1-2 IM angle was the sole criterion for radiographic success. The actual hallux valgus deformity at the MTP joint was not quantified. Significant problems were seen with transfer metatarsalgia from first ray shortening. Although we know that an increased 1-2 IM angle is important, other significant aspects of the deformity must be addressed to achieve a successful surgical outcome.

Helal[21] also reviewed his experience with operative treatment of the adolescent hallux valgus deformity. He reported on the use of eight different procedures, including the Simmonds, Golden, McBride, Modified McBride, Wilson, Peabody, Mitchel, and Joplin osteotomies. In his initial review, treatment of the deformity was met with poor results. He described the most common reason for poor results as metatarsalgia associated with a dorsal shift or tilt of the first metatarsal. He recommended that surgical treatment be performed in the early rather than late teens. Although the DMAA had not yet been described, he noted that "any attempt to realign the hallux on the metatarsal will alter the congruity of the joint surfaces and may cause degeneration of the articular cartilage with subsequent pain and stiffness." This last comment shows significant insight into a concept that had not yet been fully described and illustrates the need to correct the DMAA to realign and maintain congruity of the first MTP joint.

The surgical treatment of adolescent bunions with congruent joints must address all deformities, including the 1-2 IM angle, hallux valgus angle, DMAA, and hallux valgus interphalangeus angle. The key to the juvenile bunion lies with the DMAA. Most of the described operations achieve an intra-articular correction of the deformity by realigning the subluxated hallux back on the metatarsal head. With an increased DMAA, however, the necessity of an extra-articular osteotomy becomes apparent.[21,50–55] An intra-articular repair in these cases leads to an incongruent joint that results in pain and stiffness or early recurrence.[21,50–52] By performing an extra-articular repair, the DMAA is corrected, which allows for correction of the deformity with maintenance of joint congruity. The DMAA correction must be factored into the correction of the other parameters.

BIPLANAR CHEVRON/AKIN DOUBLE OSTEOTOMY

The distal chevron osteotomy was described by Corless[56] and Austin and Leventen[57] and is one of the most commonly used operations for the treatment of the mild to moderate hallux valgus deformity. It may be combined with an Akin osteotomy as a double osteotomy in cases with significant hallux valgus interphalangeus or a residual pronation deformity.[58] The increase in the DMAA seen with a congruent deformity presents an additional challenge. Mann[59] described the addition of a biplanar component to distal the chevron osteotomy to correct the DMAA (**Fig. 3**A, B).

Nery and colleagues[60] reported on their experience using the biplanar distal chevron osteotomy. Clinical and radiographic data were reviewed in more than 60 patients (100 feet). They noted a decrease in DMAA from 15° to 5° along with a reduction in the hallux valgus angle from 25° to 14° and 1-2 IM angle from 12° to 8°. Ninety

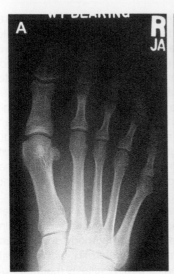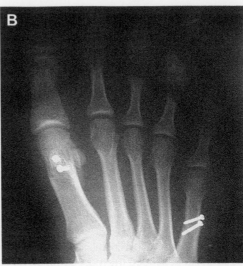

Fig. 3. (*A*) Preoperative radiograph of a 15-year-old girl with a mild congruent hallux valgus deformity. (*B*) Postoperative radiograph after biplanar chevron bunionectomy. The patient also underwent surgical correction of the bunionette deformity with a Coughlin diaphyseal osteotomy.

percent of patients were satisfied with the results of the procedure. Chou and colleagues[61] also reported on the use of the biplanar distal chevron osteotomy. They studied the results of this procedure in 14 patients, for a total of 17 feet. The correction of angular deformities was significant but less than that seen in Nery's[60] report. They achieved a DMAA correction from 16° to 9° while noting a hallux valgus angle reduction from 22° to 18° and 1-2 IM angle reduction from 11° to 9°. Although the hallux valgus and 1-2 IM angle reductions were modest, the most significant was the 7° decrease in the DMAA.

The vascular supply to the first metatarsal head has been reported as a concern with the use of distal osteotomies.[62–66] Malal and colleagues[67] studied the vascular supply to the first metatarsal head in cadaveric specimens. They found that the plantar-lateral corner of the metatarsal neck was the predominant site of vascular supply to the metatarsal head. Based on this finding, they recommended making a longer plantar limb when performing the chevron osteotomy.

Resch and colleagues[68] studied the effects of the distal chevron osteotomy with and without a lateral release with radiographs and scintigraphy. Although scintigraphy did show evidence of decreased blood supply in four metatarsal heads in the initial postoperative period, all of these lesions progressed to healing. At final follow-up averaging 19 months, no clinical or radiographic evidence of osteonecrosis was evident in either group.

More recently, Kuhn and colleagues[69] examined the blood supply to the first metatarsal head during various stages of a distal chevron bunionectomy with use of a Doppler probe. They showed a 71% total decrease in blood supply to the metatarsal head when the chevron osteotomy was combined with an adductor tenotomy. Of interest, the medial capsulotomy caused the greatest decrease in blood supply with 45%. The addition of the adductor tenotomy only added an additional 13% decrease in blood flow to the metatarsal head. No cases of avascular necrosis were noted in this series, and they concluded that the combination of an adductor tenotomy with chevron bunionectomy was safe and desirable to prevent the recurrence of deformity.

FIRST METATARSAL DOUBLE AND TRIPLE OSTEOTOMY

With moderate and severe deformities, the use of double and triple osteotomies of the first ray is indicated. This multiple osteotomy technique was developed in response to the high recurrence rate noted in the treatment of congruent hallux valgus deformities. The concept behind the use of multiple osteotomies is to correct each component of the deformity. This includes a proximal metatarsal osteotomy or medial cuneiform osteotomy to correct the 1-2 IM angle, a distal metatarsal osteotomy to correct the DMAA, and the addition of a phalangeal Akin osteotomy to correct a hallux valgus interphalangeus or residual pronation deformity (**Fig. 4**A, B).

Coughlin[16] studied the characteristics and surgical results in the adolescent population. He noted that a significantly increased DMAA and hallux valgus deformity was present in patients with onset of deformity before 10 years of age. Patients younger than 10 years at the age of onset had an average DMAA of 14.9°, compared with 8.9° with onset older than 10 years. He showed no recurrence of deformity in juvenile patients treated with a double metatarsal osteotomy and indicated that the double osteotomy was the most successful procedure for the correction of the congruent hallux valgus deformity. Coughlin[30] then studied the relationship of the DMAA in men with hallux valgus deformity. Men are much less likely than women to be affected with the hallux valgus deformity, with most reports showing that women constitute more than 90% of the patient population.[4–6,31,49,58] Coughlin noted that 37% of men undergoing hallux valgus correction had a nonsubluxated or congruent joint, which is significantly higher than the 7% and 9% observed in women as reported in other series.[3,37] He noted that with use of a distal soft-tissue procedure with proximal metatarsal osteotomy, the postoperative hallux valgus angle mirrored the DMAA. He concluded that a congruent hallux valgus deformity is resistant to correction using an intra-articular repair, which shows the importance of the DMAA in surgical planning of the hallux valgus deformity. The use of an intra-articular repair with a congruent joint

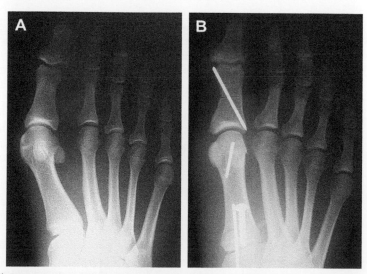

Fig. 4. (*A*) Preoperative radiograph of 16-year-old girl with a moderate congruent hallux valgus deformity. (*B*) Postoperative radiograph after first ray triple osteotomy. A 3.5-mm cortical screw with 0.062 Kirschner wire was used to fixate the proximal metatarsal osteotomy as her physes were closed.

leads to either early recurrence or a noncongruent joint with decreased motion and arthritic changes (**Fig. 5**).

Aronson and colleagues[70] also reported on their experience with the double first metatarsal osteotomy. Previous reports have shown that postoperative stiffness at the first MTP joint is a major predictor of patient satisfaction after adolescent hallux valgus repair.[22,54,71] They described a modification of the double osteotomy described by Peterson and Newman[55] using a medial plate for osteotomy fixation. In their series of 18 feet in 16 patients, they noted recurrence in 3 feet in 2 patients. These recurrences were retrospectively related to undercorrection. Clinically, however, all patients reported no pain or functional limitations.

Johnson and colleagues[72] reported on their use of the first metatarsal double osteotomy in the treatment of the adolescent hallux valgus deformity. In their series of 10 feet in 7 patients with an average follow-up of 27 months, there were no recurrences. The subjective results reported by the patients were closely related to the motion at the first MTP joint. They also concluded that the presence of open physes is not a contraindication to surgical treatment. Their article showed the importance of treating the congruent hallux valgus deformity with an extra-articular repair.

Coughlin and Carlson[73] evaluated the results of double and triple first ray osteotomies for the treatment of hallux valgus deformities with an increased DMAA. The study included 21 feet (18 patients) with an average follow-up of 33 months. Correction of the hallux valgus and 1-2 IM angles was 23° and 9°, respectively. The DMAA improved from 23° preoperatively to 9 degrees postoperatively. There were no recurrences. Twelve of the 18 patients in this study underwent surgical correction before 20 years of age. The authors noted that although a congruent deformity is more likely to present in the second decade of life, it also may present as an "adult deformity." The orthopedic surgeon must be aware of this so that the appropriate surgical procedure can be chosen.

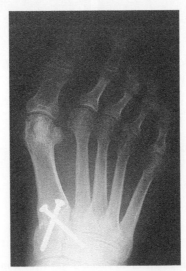

Fig. 5. Radiograph of a 45-year-old woman with a recurrent hallux valgus deformity. Despite a successful Lapidus fusion, early recurrence ensued. The magnitude of her postoperative deformity is equal to that of the increased DMAA.

There is significant controversy in the literature regarding the surgical treatment of patients with open physes. Reports of increased recurrence[4,20,21,24,25,28,53,74] and no contraindication abound.[18,75–77] Coughlin[16] demonstrated that the correction achieved in patients undergoing surgical repair with an open physis was not diminished when compared with patients undergoing surgery with closed physes. Although there is certainly no rush to perform surgery in skeletally immature patients, the presence of open physes is not a contraindication to surgical intervention (**Fig. 6**A, B).

Surgical correction of the juvenile hallux valgus deformity with a lateral hemiepiphyseodesis has been advocated in several reports.[17,78–83] Most recently, Davids and colleagues[78] published their experience with the procedure. In their group of 11 patients treated with more than 2 years of growth remaining, a significant correction was achieved in only 50% of cases. Although statistical significance was found, a look at the numerical values is less encouraging. With a 4-year follow-up, the average hallux valgus and 1-2 IM angle corrections were 2.32° (15.45°–13.13°) and 3.45° (34.64°–31.18°), respectively. Despite these small deformity corrections, the authors concluded that this technique is a viable treatment option. We feel that such a small correction in deformity, although statistically significant, is suboptimal and do not advocate its use.

AUTHORS' PREFERRED TECHNIQUE

An esmark is used to exsanguinate the extremity and is used as a tourniquet. A distal medial incision is first made over the first MTP joint. Sharp dissection is performed down to the first MTP joint capsule. The dorsal medial cutaneous nerve is protected during the dissection. It is important to note that this nerve tends to rest in a more midline position compared with the subluxated hallux valgus deformity, in which the nerve tends to lie in a more dorsal position. An inverted L-shaped capsulotomy is made to release the proximal and dorsal aspect of the MTP joint capsule exposing

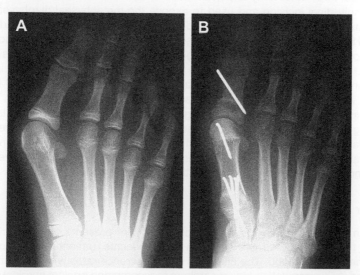

Fig. 6. (*A*) Preoperative radiograph of a 12-year-old girl with a moderate congruent hallux valgus deformity. (*B*) Postoperative radiograph after first ray triple osteotomy. Fixation was achieved with 0.062 Kirschner wires alone at all osteotomy sites as her physes were open.

the medial eminence. An oscillating saw is used to resect the medial eminence starting approximately 2 mm medial to the sagittal sulcus. The remaining edges are beveled with a rongeur. A lateral release, either intra-articular or through a separate incision, is not performed out of concern for the blood supply to the first metatarsal head.

Attention is then turned to the extra-articular correction. A medial closing wedge Reverdin osteotomy is made at the metaphyseal/diaphyseal region just proximal to the sesamoids.[84–86] Care is taken not to overly penetrate the lateral cortex so as not to compromise the circulation to the first metatarsal head. The osteotomy is closed and fixated with one or two 0.062-inch Kirschner wires placed in a dorsal-distal to plantar-proximal direction. The Kirschner wire is then bent and cut to allow for later removal. By performing this osteotomy first, the DMAA is corrected and attention can be turned to correcting the deformity, as would be done in the case of a subluxated hallux valgus deformity.

A dorsal longitudinal incision is made proximally centered over the proximal first metatarsal. The dissection is performed medial to the extensor hallucis longus tendon, which is retracted laterally. A crescentic osteotomy is made 1.0 to 1.3 cm distal to the first metatarsocuneiform joint. Care is taken not to violate an open physis if present. If present, the osteotomy is made an additional 5 mm distal to avoid the open physis. The osteotomy is displaced 2 to 4 mm laterally to reduce the 1-2 IM angle. It is then fixated with a 0.062-inch Kirschner wire and 3.5-mm cortical screw placed in lag fashion. If an open physis is present, the osteotomy is fixated with three to four 0.062-inch Kirschner wires.

After fixation of both osteotomies, the medial capsule is repaired. A 2-mm dorsal-to-plantar drill hole is made in the distal metatarsal metaphysis and is used to repair the capsule back to bone. The medial capsulorraphy is then completed. Intraoperative fluoroscopy is used to ensure reduction of all radiographic parameters and guard against overcorrection leading to hallux varus.

If there is a significant hallux valgus interphalangeus or residual pronation deformity, a phalangeal Akin osteotomy is performed. A 2-cm distal extension is made to the medial longitudinal incision and used to expose the metaphyseal/diaphyseal region of the proximal phalanx. A medial-based closing wedge osteotomy is made 3 to 4 mm distal to the proximal phalangeal physeal scar. If the physis is open, intraoperative fluoroscopy is used to identify the physis before the osteotomy is made. The size of the medial wedge to be removed depends on the magnitude of the hallux valgus interphalangeus angle. The osteotomy is closed and then fixated with one to two 0.062-inch Kirschner wires, and intraoperative fluoroscopy is used to confirm alignment. The incisions are irrigated and closed in layers. A gauze and tape toe-spica dressing is applied and changed every 10 days over an 8-week period. Weight-bearing is allowed on the heel and lateral aspect of the foot in a postoperative stiff-soled shoe. The Akin pins are removed at 3 to 4 weeks, with the remaining hardware being removed at 6 weeks. Full activity and running are not permitted until 3 months postoperatively.

SUMMARY

The treatment of hallux valgus with a congruent joint presents a unique challenge. Although the deformity is more common in adolescents, patients may also present for treatment in adulthood. The history of high recurrence rates with standard procedures seen in this population led researchers to recommend against surgical intervention in the young. We now know that the high failure rate was not inherent to the patient population but rather was the result of a lack of appreciation of the deformity. The increased DMAA is a critical component of the deformity that must be addressed for surgical success. Extra-articular repair using double and triple first ray osteotomies corrects all components of the deformity and has been shown to have success rates similar to that seen in the treatment of the more common subluxated deformity. Clinicians must be aware of the DMAA in all patients who present for treatment of hallux valgus to optimize the success of surgical correction.

REFERENCES

1. Kelikian H. Hallux valgus, allied deformities of the forefoot and metatarsalgia. Philadelphia: WB Saunders; 1965. p. 27–68, 241.
2. Myerson M. Foot and ankle disorders, hallux valgus. Philadelphia: WB Suanders; 1999. p. 213–89.
3. Coughlin M, Jones C. Hallux valgus: demographics, etiology, and radiographic assessment. Foot Ankle Int 2007;28:759–77.
4. Bonney G, MacNab I. Hallux valgus and hallux rigidus: a critical survey of operative results. J Bone Joint Surg Br 1952;34:366–85.
5. Glynn M, Dunlop J, FitzPatrick D. The Mitchell distal metatarsal osteotomy for hallux valgus. J Bone Joint Surg Br 1980;62:188–91.
6. Hardy R, Clapham J. Observations on hallux valgus. J Bone Joint Surg Br 1951; 33:376–91.
7. Barnicot NA, Hardy RH. The position of the hallux in West Africans. J Anat 1955; 89:355–61.
8. Engle ET, Morton DJ. Notes of foot disorders among natives of the Belgian Congo. J Bone Joint Surg 1931;13:311.
9. James C. Foot prints and feet of natives of Soloman Islands. Lancet 1939;2:1390.
10. Maclennan R. Prevalence of hallux valgus in a Neolithic New Guinea population. Lancet 1966;1:1398–400.
11. Shine IB. Incidence of hallux valgus in a partially shoe-wearing community. Br Med J 1965;26:1648–50.
12. Wells LH. The foot of the South African native. Am J Phys Anthropol 1931;15:185.
13. Sim-Fook L, Hodgson AR. A comparison of foot forms among the non-shoe and shoe-wearing Chinese population. J Bone Joint Surg Am 1958;40:1058–62.
14. Kato T, Watanabe S. The etiology of hallux valgus in Japan. Clin Orthop 1981;157: 78–81.
15. Canale P, Aronsson D, Lamont R, et al. The Mitchell procedure for the treatment of adolescent hallux valgus. J Bone Joint Surg Am 1993;75:1610–8.
16. Coughlin M. Juvenile hallux valgus: etiology and treatment. Foot Ankle Int 1995; 16:682–97.
17. Ellis V. A method of correcting metatarsus primus varus. J Bone Joint Surg Br 1951;33:415–7.
18. Geissle A, Stanton R. Surgical treatment of adolescent hallux valgus. J Pediatr Orthop 1990;10:642–8.
19. Grosio J. Juvenile hallux valgus: a conservative approach to treatment. J Bone Joint Surg Am 1992;74:1367–74.
20. Halebian J, Gaines S. Juvenile hallux valgus. J Foot Surg 1983;22:290–3.
21. Helal B. Surgery for adolescent hallux valgus. Clin Orthop 1981;157:50–63.
22. Luba R, Rosman M. Bunions in children: treatment with a modified Mitchell osteotomy. J Pediatr Orthop 1984;4:44–7.
23. Mahan K, Jacko J. Juvenile hallux valgus with compensated metatarsus adductus: a case report. J Am Podiatr Med Assoc 1991;81:525–30.

24. McHale K, McKay D. Bunions in a child: conservative versus surgical management. J Musculoskel Med 1986;3:56–62.
25. Meehan P. Adolescent bunion. Instr Course Lect 1982;31:262–4.
26. Mitchell C, Fleming J, Allen R, et al. Osteotomy-bunionectomy for hallux valgus. J Bone Joint Surg Am 1958;40:41–58.
27. Scranton P. Adolescent bunions: diagnosis and management. Pediatr Ann 1982; 11:518–20.
28. Scranton P, Zuckerman J. Bunion surgery in the adolescent: results of surgical treatment. J Pediatr Orthop 1984;1:39–43.
29. Coughlin MJ, Saltzman CL, Nunley JA. Angular measurements in the evaluation of hallux valgus deformities: a report of the ad hoc committee of the American Orthopaedic Foot and Ankle Society on angular measurements. Foot Ankle Int 2002;23:68–74.
30. Coughlin M. Hallux valgus in men: effect of the distal metatarsal articular angle on hallux valgus correction. Foot Ankle Int 1997;18:463–70.
31. Wu K. Wu's bunionectomy: a clinical analysis of 150 personal cases. J Foot Surg 1992;31:288–97.
32. Coughlin M, Freund E. The reliability of angular measurements in hallux valgus deformities. Foot Ankle Int 2001;22:369–79.
33. Saltzman C, Brandser E, Berbaum K, et al. Reliability of standard foot radiographic measurements. Foot Ankle Int 1994;15:661–5.
34. Vittetoe D, Saltzman C, Krieg J, et al. Reliability and validity of distal metatarsal articular angle. Foot Ankle Int 1994;15:541–7.
35. Chi TD, Davitt J, Younger A, et al. Intra- and inter-observer reliability of the distal metatarsal articular angle in adult hallux valgus. Foot Ankle Int 2002;23:722–6.
36. Richardson G, Graves S, McClure J, et al. First metatarsal head-shaft angle: a method of determination. Foot Ankle 1993;14:181–5.
37. Piggott H. The natural history of hallux valgus in adolescence and early adult life. J Bone Joint Surg Br 1960;42:749–60.
38. Hawkins F, Mitchell C, Hedrick D. Correction of hallux valgus by metatarsal osteotomy. J Bone Joint Surg 1945;27:387–94.
39. Jones A. Hallux valgus in the adolescent. Proc R Soc Med 1948;41:392–3.
40. Ball J, Sullivan J. Treatment of the juvenile bunion by Mitchell osteotomy. Orthopedics 1985;8:1249–52.
41. Pontious J, Mahan K, Carter S. Characteristics of adolescent hallux abducto valgus: a retrospective study. J Am Podiatr Med Assoc 1994;84:208–18.
42. Kalen V, Brecher A. Relationship between adolescent bunions and flat feet. Foot Ankle 1988;8:331–6.
43. Amarnek D, Jacobs A, Oloff L. Adolescent hallux valgus: its etiology and surgical management. J Foot Ankle Surg 1985;24:54–61.
44. Greenberg G. Relationship of hallux abductus angle and first metatarsal angle to severity of pronation. J Am Podiatr Med Assoc 1979;69:29–34.
45. Inman V. Hallux valgus: a review of etiologic factors. Orthop Clin North Am 1974; 5:59–66.
46. Trott A. Hallux valgus in adolescents. Instr Course Lect 1972;21:262–8.
47. Coughlin MJ, Jones CP. Hallux valgus and first ray mobility: a prospective study. J Bone Joint Surg Am 2007;89:1887–98.
48. Kilmartin T, Wallace W. The significance of pes planus in juvenile hallux valgus. Foot Ankle 1992;13:53–6.
49. Carr C, Boyd B. Correctional osteotomy for metatsus primus varus and hallux valgus. J Bone Joint Surg Am 1968;50:1353–67.

50. Amarnek D, Mollica A, Jacobs A, et al. A statistical analysis on the reliability of the proximal articular set angle. J Foot Surg 1986;25:39–42.
51. Cholmeley J. Hallux valgus in adolescents. Proc R Soc Med 1958;51:903–6.
52. Coughlin M, Bordelon R, Johnson K, et al. President's forum: evaluation and treatment of juvenile hallux valgus. Contemp Orthop 1990;21:169–203.
53. Coughlin M, Mann R. The pathophysiology of the juvenile bunion. Instr Course Lect 1987;36:123–36.
54. Das De S. Distal metatarsal osteotomy for adolescent hallux valgus. J Pediatr Orthop 1984;4:32–8.
55. Peterson H, Newman S. Adolescent bunion deformity treated with double osteotomy and longitudinal pin fixation of the first ray. J Pediatr Orthop 1993; 13:80–4.
56. Corless JR. A modification of the Mitchell procedure. J Bone Joint Surg 1976;55/58B:138.
57. Austin DW, Leventen EO. A new osteotomy for hallux valgus: a horizontally directed "V" displacement osteotomy of the metatarsal head for hallux valgus and primus varus. Clin Orthop 1981;157:25–30.
58. Mitchell L, Baxter D. The chevron-Akin double osteotomy for correction of hallux valgus. Foot Ankle 1991;12:7–14.
59. Mann RA. Disorders of the first metatarsophalangeal joint. J Am Acad Orthop Surg 1995;3:34–43.
60. Nery C, Barroco R, Ressio C. Biplanar chevron osteotomy. Foot Ankle Int 2002;23: 792–8.
61. Chou L, Mann R, Casillas M. Biplanar chevron osteotomy. Foot Ankle Int 1998;19: 579–84.
62. Horne G, Tanzer T, Ford M. Chevron osteotomy for the treatment of hallux valgus. Clin Orthop 1984;183:32–6.
63. Kinnard P, Gordon D. A comparison between chevron and Mitchell osteotomies for hallux valgus. Foot Ankle 1984;4:241–3.
64. Jones KJ, Feiwell LA, Freedman EL, et al. The effect of chevron osteotomy with lateral capsular release on the blood supply to the first metatarsal head. J Bone Joint Surg Am 1995;77:197–204.
65. Mann RA. Complications associated with the chevron osteotomy. Foot Ankle 1982;3:125–9.
66. Meier PJ, Kenzora JE. The risks and benefits of distal first metatarsal osteotomies. Foot Ankle 1985;6:7–17.
67. Malal JJ, Shaw-Dunn J, Kumas CS. Blood supply to the first metatarsal head and vessels at risk with a chevron osteotomy. J Bone Joint Surg Am 2007;89: 2018–22.
68. Resch S, Stenstrom A, Gustafson T. Circulatory disturbance of the first metatarsal head after Chevron osteotomy as shown by bone scintigraphy. Foot Ankle Int 1992;13:137–42.
69. Kuhn MA, Lippert FG, Phipps MJ, et al. Blood flow to the metatarsal head after chevron bunionectomy. Foot Ankle Int 2005;26:526–9.
70. Aronson J, Nguyen LL, Aronson EA. Early results of the modified Peterson bunion procedure for adolescent hallux valgus. J Pediatr Orthop 2001;21:65–9.
71. McDonald MG, Stevens DB. Modified Mitchell bunionectomy for management of adolescent hallux valgus. Clin Orthop 1996;332:163–9.
72. Johnson AE, Georgopoulos G, Erickson MA, et al. Treatment of adolescent hallux valgus with the first metatarsal double osteotomy: the Denver experience. J Pediatr Orthop 2004;24(4):358–62.

73. Coughlin MJ, Carlson RE. Treatment of hallux valgus with an increased distal metatarsal articular angle: evaluation of double and triple first ray osteotomies. Foot Ankle Int 1999;20:762–70.
74. Mann R, Coughlin M. Hallux valgus: etiology, anatomy, treatment, and surgical considerations. Clin Orthop 1981;157:31–41.
75. Gerbert J. The indications and techniques for utilizing preoperative templates in podiatric surgery. J Am Podiatr Med Assoc 1979;69:139–48.
76. Simmonds F, Menelaus M. Hallux valgus in adolescents. J Bone Joint Surg Br 1960;42:761–8.
77. Andreacchio A, Origo C, Rocca G. Early results of the modified Simmonds-Mene-laus procedure for adolescent hallux valgus. J Pediatr Orthop 2002;22:375–9.
78. Davids JR, McBrayer D, Blackhurst DW. Juvenile hallux valgus deformity: surgical management by lateral hemiepiphyseodesis of the great toe metatarsal. J Pediatr Orthop 2007;27:826–30.
79. Fox IM, Smith SD. Juvenile bunion correction by epiphysiodesis of the first meta-tarsal. J Am Podiatry Assoc 1983;73:448–55.
80. Nelson JP. Mechanical arrestment of bone growth for the correction of pedal deformities. J Foot Surg 1981;20:14–6.
81. Ribotsky BM, Nazarian S, Scheuller HC. Epiphysiodesis of the first metatarsal with cancellous allograft. J Am Podiatr Med Assoc 1993;83:263–6.
82. Seiberg M, Green R, Green D. Epiphysiodesis in juvenile hallux abductovalgus: a preliminary retrospective study. J Am Podiatr Med Assoc 1994;84:225–36.
83. Sheridan LE. Correction of juvenile hallux valgus deformity associated with meta-tarsus primus adductus using epiphysiodesis technique. Clin Podiatr Med Surg 1987;4:63–74.
84. Reverdin J. De la deviation en dehors du gros orteil et de son traitement chirur-gical. Trans Int Med Congr 1881;2:408–12 [in French].
85. Peabody D. Surgical care of hallux valgus. J Bone Joint Surg 1931;13:273–82.
86. Hohmann G. Der hallux valgus und die uebrigen zchenverkruemmungen. Egerb Chir Orthop 1925;18:308–48 [in German].

Non-Neuropathic Midfoot Multiplanar Deformity: Surgical Strategies for Reconstruction

Bryan D. Den Hartog, MD[a,c,]*, David B. Kay, MD[b]

KEYWORDS

- Midfoot • Deformity • Multiplanar • Reconstruction • Flatfoot

Painful collapse of the midfoot medial longitudinal arch can occur as a complication of rheumatoid or osteoarthritis of the midfoot or trauma to the talus, cuneiforms, or Lisfranc joint.[1,2] Other causes include progressive tendinopathy with rupture of the plantar fascia, spring ligament, and Charcot osteoarthropathy.

The most common multiplanar deformity of the midfoot is pes planovalgus. Clinically, the flatfoot is characterized by a depressed or absent medial longitudinal arch accompanied by forefoot abduction and, in some cases, by supination of the forefoot and valgus angulation of the hindfoot.[3,4]

For those patients who fail nonoperative treatment, the goal of reconstruction should be to establish a painless plantigrade foot that is free from bony prominences and able to accommodate regular shoes. There are various reports of techniques that allow this type of stable deformity correction at the time of arthrodesis.[1,5,6]

This article reviews the reconstructive strategies for correction of deformity and fusion of the painful arthritic joints. A stepwise surgical approach is recommended for reproducible correction and midfoot fusion in patients with arthritis combined with a multiplanar deformity. We will focus on the principles of reconstruction of the planovalgus deformity in the non-neuropathic patient using compression plates for a stable construct fixation.

[a] Black Hills Orthopedic & Spine Center, PO Box 6850, Rapid City, SD 57709-6850, USA
[b] Northeast Ohio University College of Medicine, 4209 Street, Route 44, P.O. Box 95, Rootstown, OH 44272, USA
[c] Sanford School of Medicine, 640 Flormann Street, Suite 120, Rapid City, SD 57701, USA
* Corresponding author.
E-mail address: bryandenhartog@bhosc.com (B.D. Den Hartog).

Foot Ankle Clin N Am 14 (2009) 383–392
doi:10.1016/j.fcl.2009.06.004
1083-7515/09/$ – see front matter © 2009 Elsevier Inc. All rights reserved.

CLINICAL PRESENTATION
Pain

Painful arthritis frequently follows midfoot fractures and fracture-dislocations. The arthritis is commonly accompanied by residual foot deformity, most commonly a planus or planovalgus deformity, but cavus deformities have been reported.[5,7]

Secondary causes of pain include lateral hindfoot impingement in the sinus tarsi as the anterior process of the calcaneus abuts against the fibula as the hindfoot goes into severe valgus. The patient often reports foot fatigue with standing and walking.

Progressive Deformity

With collapse of the midfoot joints due to degenerative arthritis, trauma, or rupture of the posterior tibial tendon, the medial longitudinal arch begins to drop in a plantigrade direction, initiating progressive structural changes in the foot that lead to the pes planovalgus deformity (**Fig. 1**).[8,9] Exaggerated pressure points can cause painful calluses under the midfoot. The deformity can cause excessive shoe wear along the medial heel and arch with breakdown of the heel counter.

Gait Abnormalities

As the flatfoot develops, the gait becomes apropulsive, so instead of having a fluid, continuous stride with a reciprocating gait, the patient has a halting, so-called "stop-and-start" gait because of ineffective push-off.[10] An altered gait can cause excess strain on the knee, hip, and back.

DIAGNOSIS
Physical Examination

It is imperative to evaluate the entire lower extremity for deformity. The problem may not be limited to the midfoot and may involve excessive genu varus or valgus, hindfoot valgus, or fixed forefoot supination. To most accurately assess foot and ankle position, it is helpful to have the patient stand. Look for asymmetric collapse of the medial longitudinal arch, forefoot abduction, or hindfoot varus or valgus. Locate bony prominences at the apex of the deformity and any associated skin breakdown or callusing. Assess for excessive or compensatory tightening of the gastrocnemius or Achilles tendons.

Radiographs

Standing anteroposterior and lateral views demonstrate the location of the midfoot deformity and the specific joints involved (**Fig. 2**A). The radiographs allow identification of the apex of deformity for operative planning and identification of those joints

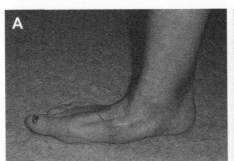
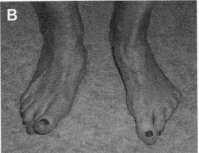

Fig. 1. (*A* and *B*) A collapsed midfoot after a fracture dislocation of the Lisfranc joint.

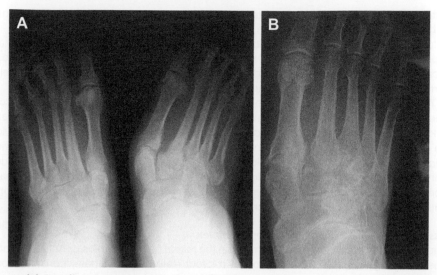

Fig. 2. (A) Standing anteroposterior foot radiograph showing collapsed apex of the right midfoot at the medial side of the Lisfranc joint. (B) Anteroposterior radiograph of a foot with Lisfranc joint involvement with arthrosis also at the naviculocuneiform joints.

in the midfoot that may be involved in the arthritic process (ie, the intercuneiform joints) (**Fig. 2B**). Failure to identify and address all the involved joints may result in persistent midfoot pain postoperatively.

Standing lateral view

The standing lateral radiograph identifies the segment or segments of collapse of the medial column, which can occur in through the Lisfranc joint (**Fig. 3**) or elsewhere in the midfoot, including the naviculocuneiform and talonavicular joints.

Strategy for Reconstruction

When a patient has persistent debilitating pain despite proper nonoperative treatment measures, such as shoe modification or orthotics, and a multiplanar deformity is present, a step-wise approach to surgical correction is important to improve chances of achieving the goal of a painless, plantigrade foot.[6] When performing a fusion or

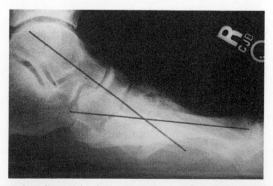

Fig. 3. Standing lateral radiograph demonstrating posttraumatic collapse of the medial column of the midfoot with the apex of deformity at the Lisfranc joint and disruption of the talo–first metatarsal line.

osteotomy, it is essential to re-create normal alignment of the talo–first metatarsal line in both the axial and sagittal planes.

Identify where the deformity is located and in what direction (usually dorsal-lateral biplanar). Correction is performed at the apex of the deformity. This apex may be located at multiple areas in the midfoot (ie, naviculocuneiform and metatarsocuneiform) or at a single level (ie, metatarsocuneiform only).

The midfoot deformity cannot be addressed in isolation. Careful consideration of knee, hindfoot, and forefoot alignment and flexibility of the gastrocsoleus complex is key to a successful surgical outcome. In general, the corrective procedures should be done sequentially starting proximal to distal to assure proper foot alignment. The sequence recommended is as follows: (1) improve flexibility of the gastrocsoleus complex; (2) correct hindfoot malalignment; (3) address forefoot supination or pronation; (4) address forefoot abduction or adduction; (5) address rocker bottom deformities; (6) address multiplanar deformities.

Assess flexibility of the gastrocsoleus complex

Though there is not universal agreement on the role of gastrocnemius or Achilles tightness in the genesis or exacerbation of midfoot deformity and pain, consideration should be given to either a gastrocnemius slide or percutaneous Achilles lengthening if there is severe limitation of ankle dorsiflexion when the hindfoot is held in neutral. Excessive tightness may cause undo stress on the reconstructed midfoot once it has healed.

Check hindfoot alignment

Heel varus deformity is corrected using a closing wedge (Dwyer) osteotomy with lateral translation of the calcaneus. The osteotomy can be secured with a cannulated screw (**Fig. 4**), compression staple, or compression plate. Excessive hindfoot valgus is corrected with a medial displacement osteotomy with 1 to 1.5 cm of translation and secured with an intramedullary-extramedullary device (**Fig. 5**) or cannulated screw.

Address forefoot supination or pronation

If the forefoot is supinated or pronated, the distal part of the foot is rotated to neutral through a transverse osteotomy either through the medial column only or through the whole midfoot if the arthrosis or deformity extends across the entire midfoot. This derotation may be done through the transverse tarsal, Lisfranc joint, or the intertarsal region, depending on where the arthritic joints and deformity are located. Again, the

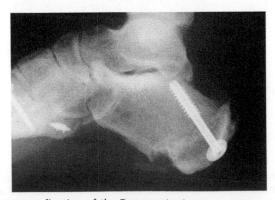

Fig. 4. Compression screw fixation of the Dwyer osteotomy.

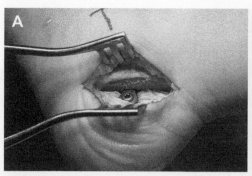
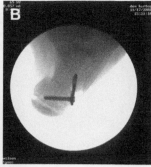

Fig. 5. (A) Fixation using the intramedullary-extramedullary fixation with the calcaneus translated 1 to 1.5 mm medially. (B) An intraoperative axial radiograph showing the medial displacement with purposeful varus tilt of the tuberosity to move the heel contact point further medially.

goal is to establish a plantigrade foot with a physiologic weight-bearing tripod between the heel contact point and the first and fifth metatarsal heads.

Address adducted or abducted forefoot

Correction of deformity through the axial plane is performed either by shortening of the medial column or lengthening of the lateral column. For mild to moderate deformities, we have found that fusion of the affected midfoot joints with a resultant moderate shortening of the medial column is adequate to reestablish normal alignment of the medial column (**Fig. 6**). However, in those patients with severe biplanar deformity, re-creation of the talo–first metatarsal line requires both an osteotomy to correct rotational deformity and the use of medial wedging to obtain the desired plantigrade foot. The depth of the wedge cut depends on the severity of deformity and extent of the arthrosis. While some patients need only the medial column wedged, those with more extensive deformity may require osteotomy or wedge resection that extends across the entire width of the midfoot to obtain the needed correction (**Fig. 7**).

The closing wedge osteotomy is performed at the level of deformity (through the apex). To determine the angle of the wedge, a proximal pin can be placed perpendicular to the plane of the hindfoot. A second distal pin is placed as perpendicular as possible to the plane of the forefoot (**Fig. 8**A, B). The cuts are then made to remove

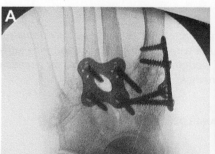
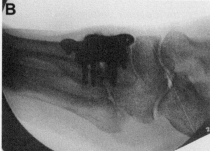

Fig. 6. Intraoperative radiographs (anteroposterior [A] and lateral [B]) showing a medial column only reconstruction.

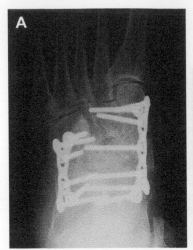

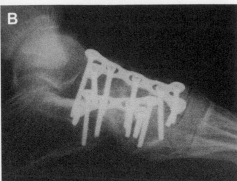

Fig. 7. (*A*) Medial and (*B*) lateral postoperative radiographs demonstrating a column reconstruction requiring derotation and wedging of the entire width of the midfoot.

the bone inside the pin boundaries (**Fig. 8**C). Rigid fixation with low-profile contoured compression plates (**Fig. 8**D, E) can maximize construct stability and reduce the chance of recurrence of deformity during the healing period.

Cannulated screws or low-profile compression plates can be used to stabilize the construct (see **Fig. 8**D, E). Some investigators suggest avoiding a fusion of the fourth and fifth metatarsal-cuneiform joint. They say that, by aligning the medial column (the talo–first metatarsal line), the lateral Lisfranc joint will be decompressed and likely not as painful.[11,12] This would lengthen the lateral column as the medial column is shortened to correct the dorsolateral deformity.[11]

Address rocker bottom deformities

After the abduction deformity has been addressed, the deformity in the sagittal plane (dorsiflexion of the forefoot) is corrected with a plantar-based closing wedge osteotomy through the same osteotomy used to correct the forefoot abduction. If a rocker bottom deformity exists at either the calcaneal cuboid and talonavicular (transverse tarsal) joints or the Lisfranc joint, a plantar or plantar medial closing wedge osteotomy is used to reconstruct the normal arch height (with reduction of the talo–first metatarsal line) and the weight-bearing tripod.

Address multiplanar deformities

Correction is achieved with all the above-mentioned principles. This may require the removal of multiple bone wedges. Again, guide wires can be used to determine angles for bone wedge removal. A combination of wedging and derotation will be necessary for correction of complex multiplanar deformities.

SURGICAL TECHNIQUE FOR MIDFOOT MULTIPLANAR DEFORMITY CORRECTION: CASE EXAMPLE

Our approach is to work proximal to distal for sequential correction of the deformity. We first consider addressing any existing tightness of the gastrocsoleus complex by performing either a gastrocnemius slide or percutaneous heel-cord lengthening. If

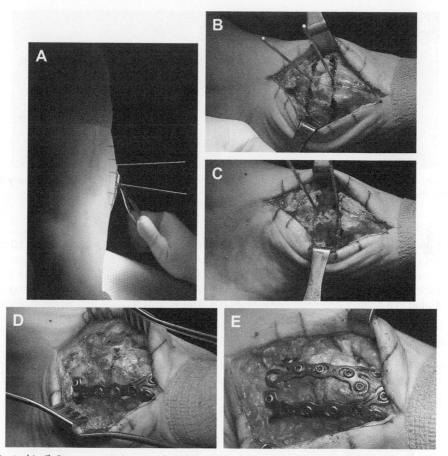

Fig. 8. (*A–C*) Convergent pins are placed to guide the wedge cuts through the apex of defor-mity. (*D* and *E*) The wedge is then removed and low-profile compression plates applied for rigid fixation of the medial column.

excessive hindfoot valgus is present, a medial displacement calcaneal osteotomy is done to place the heel in approximately 5° of valgus.

Once the hindfoot is aligned, restoration of the medial column is addressed first before addressing the other midfoot and forefoot deformities. Occasionally it will be necessary to release the peroneus longus if it prevents reduction. A full-thickness mid-foot incision is made initially to expose the dorsal, medial, and plantar aspects of the medial column. Dorsal and lateral incisions can be made to access the rest of the mid-foot if the entire width of the midfoot needs to be osteotomized or fused (**Fig. 9**). Great care is taken to protect the soft tissues with broad retractors, especially when the saw cuts for the wedges are made.

A medial wedge osteotomy, usually through the Lisfranc joint, is performed first to correct the abduction deformity. Then, if necessary, a plantar-based wedge is per-formed to adjust the arch height and reconstruct the talo–first metatarsal line (**Fig. 10**). Rotation through the osteotomy may also be necessary to correct a forefoot supination deformity. Failure to do so may result in a nonplantigrade foot.

Temporary fixation with a guide wire is used with subsequent application of cannulated compression screws and plates that provide compression and rigid fixation (**Fig. 11**).

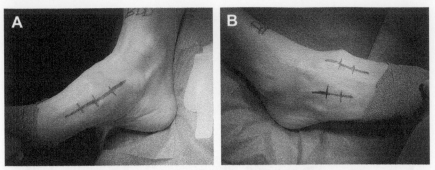

Fig. 9. (*A* and *B*) Placement of the midfoot incisions. Only the medial incision is necessary if just the medial column is reconstructed.

Postoperative Care

A bulky Jones splint is applied in the operating room. The patient is seen back in 10 to 14 days and, if the incision is healing well, a short leg cast is applied. The cast is removed at 6 weeks from surgery and radiographs taken to assess healing. If the osteotomy and fusion site appear to be uniting, a gradual increase in weight bearing is initiated in a soled Controlled Ankle Motion (CAM) Walker as pain and swelling allow.

DISCUSSION

Sangeorzan and colleagues[1] found that the deformity at the Lisfranc joint often played a role in the preoperative symptoms, abnormal shoe wear, altered gait, exaggerated

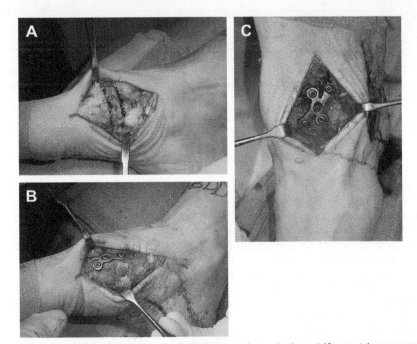

Fig. 10. (*A–C*) Sequence of wedging and derotation through the midfoot with compression plating to provide rigid fixation.

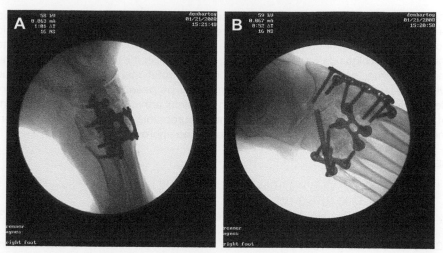

Fig. 11. (A and B) Intraoperative radiographs demonstrating reconstruction across the entire midfoot with a combination of cannulated screw and compression-plate fixation.

pressure points, and impingementlike symptoms laterally, leading to reports of foot fatigue with standing and walking. The abduction of the forefoot often led to uncovering of the talar head or prominence of the medial cuneiform, rotation of the subtalar joint, and marked hindfoot valgus, thus altering the mechanical relationships of the feet they studied. Few reports have addressed correction of deformity associated with transmetatarsal joint arthritis after trauma[1,5] and there is some controversy over whether correction of deformity is actually necessary for a good clinical outcome.[11] However, others have found that deformity reduction strongly correlated to a good outcome.[1,6] The surgical technique described by Sangeorzan[1] not only provided fusion of the painful joints but also allowed for correction of the residual deformity and demonstrated a strong correlation between deformity reduction and outcome. Reduction of deformity was the most significant predictor of good outcome in their patient group.

Horton and Olney[5] found that by gaining reduction and restoring the normal longitudinal arch of the foot, a more mechanically sound plantigrade foot was achieved and the preoperative complaints of painful callosities and inferior medial foot pain were resolved.

Toolan and colleagues[3] found that while in situ fusion of arthritic midfoot joints may be effective in relieving pain, correction of severe deformity along with fusion improved patient outcomes by eliminating bony prominences (and thus pressure points), improved shoe wear and gait, and reduced the likelihood of lateral ankle impingement from a hindfoot valgus deformity. They concluded that the relief of pain and the restoration of function achieved through effective correction of the severe pes planovalgus deformity accounted for satisfactory outcomes in 41 patients who underwent complex reconstruction for midfoot multiplanar deformity.

SUMMARY

The best patient outcomes stem from careful attention to preoperative planning where arthritic and painful joints are identified and the apex of deformity pinpointed, leading to both elimination of pain from arthrosis and correction of midfoot deformity. The reconstruction should be carried out in a sequential fashion to improve the likelihood of proper deformity correction. Routine preparation of fusion surfaces with dynamic compression plates for compression of the fusion sites can correct mild to moderate midfoot planovalgus deformities. However, to reestablish the normal alignment of the medial column, osteotomies may be needed for rotational deformities, and bone wedge resection through arthritic segments may be needed to correct angulatory deformities of the midfoot. With elimination of painful arthritic joints and achievement of proper foot alignment, the patient with non-neuropathic multiplanar midfoot deformity has a good probability of decreased pain and improved foot function.

REFERENCES

1. Sangeorzan BJ, Veith RG, Hansen ST. Salvage of Lisfranc's joint by arthrodesis. Foot Ankle 1990;10:193–200.
2. Pedowitz WJ, Kovatis P. Flatfoot in the adult. J Am Acad Orthop Surg 1995;3: 293–302.
3. Toolan BC, Sangeorzan BJ, Hansen ST. Complex reconstruction for the treatment of dorsolateral peritalar subluxation of the foot. J Bone Joint Surg Am 1999;81: 1545–60.
4. Stromont DM, Morrey BF, An KN, et al. Stability of the loaded ankle. Relation between articular restraint and primary and secondary static restraints. Am J Sports Med 1985;13:295–300.
5. Horton GA, Olney BW. Deformity and arthrodesis of the midfoot with a medial plate. Foot Ankle 1993;14:493–9.
6. Haddad SL, Myerson MS, Pell RF IV, et al. Clinical and radiographic outcome of the revision surgery for failed triple arthrodesis. Foot Ankle Int 1997;18:489–99.
7. Brunet JA, Wiley JJ. The late results of tarsometatarsal joint injuries. J Bone Joint Surg Br 1987;69:437–40.
8. Kaye RA, Jahss MH. Tibialis posterior: a review of anatomy and biomechanics in relation to support of the medial longitudinal arch. Foot Ankle 1991;11:244–7.
9. Funk DA, Cass JR, Johnson KA. Acquired adult flatfoot secondary to posterior tibial tendon pathology. J Bone Joint Surg Am 1986;68:95–102.
10. Mann RA. Acquired flatfoot in adults. Clin Orthop Relat Res 1983;181:46–51.
11. Anderson RB. Missed Lisfranc's injury. In: Nunley J, Pfeffer G, Sanders R, et al, editors. Advanced reconstruction foot and ankle. Rosemont, IL: AAOS; 2004. p. 397–400.
12. Johnson JE, Johnson KA. Dowel arthrodesis for degenerative arthritis of the tarsometatarsal (Lisfranc's) joints. Foot Ankle 1986;5:243–53.

Superconstructs in the Treatment of Charcot Foot Deformity: Plantar Plating, Locked Plating, and Axial Screw Fixation

V. James Sammarco, MD

KEYWORDS

- Charcot • Neuroarthropathy • Superconstruct • Diabetic Foot
- Limb Salvage • Arthrodesis • Axial Screw • Plantar Plate

Painless fracture dislocation associated with neuropathy in syphilitic patients was described by Jean Mation Charcot.[1] In 1936, Jordan[2] linked neuropathic fractures to diabetes. With the increasing prevalence of diabetes and neuropathy, the treatment of Charcot neuroarthropathy has become an increasingly important part of the clinician's practice. Nonoperative treatment has included total-contact cast immobilization until bony consolidation occurs, followed by accommodative bracing and footwear.[3–5] Surgery has often been reserved for patients who develop gross deformity with ulceration, and limited to simple resection of bony prominences.[6–10] Unsatisfactory outcomes in patients who have grossly unstable dislocations in the midfoot and increased instability following bony resection have led to changes of treatment protocols for neuropathic deformity.[11–24] The diabetic patient commonly has comorbid conditions involving the lower extremities, including peripheral neuropathy, peripheral vascular disease, and immune impairment. These conditions worsen with time, making late reconstruction challenging. These issues combined with progressive bony deformity and resorption that may accompany neuroarthropathy have led to advocating surgical intervention earlier in the disease process.[23]

The long-term goals for operative and nonoperative treatment are to achieve a stable, plantigrade functional foot that is resistant to ulceration, to prevent amputation, to improve performance in activities of daily living, and to allow the use of nonprescription footwear. Chronic dislocation and soft tissue contracture often require significant bony resection at surgery to restore alignment. Midfoot arthrodesis with

Cincinnati Sports Medicine and Orthopaedic Center, 10663 Montgomery Road, Cincinnati, OH 45242, USA
E-mail address: vjsammarco@csmoc.com

Foot Ankle Clin N Am 14 (2009) 393–407
doi:10.1016/j.fcl.2009.04.004

foot.theclinics.com

bony resection and osteotomy is a technique considered appropriate for early treat-ment of this deformity; however, loss of initial surgical correction and high rates of nonunion still remain common sequelae.[3,9,15,17,20] Poor bone quality, neuropathy, poor vascularity, and impaired nutrition of glycosylated tissue in diabetic patients all delay healing of the arthrodesis. Standard fixation techniques are often inadequate to maintain alignment postoperatively. In addition, patients who have neuropathy frequently have difficulty complying with long periods of non–weight bearing needed to achieve arthrodesis.[19,22,25] Previously described techniques include fixation with dorsal or plantar plates, crossed lag screws, fixation with axial screws from the talus and calcaneus, and external fixation.[12,14,21,22,26]

CLASSIFICATION

Multiple classification systems have been proposed to describe the deformities asso-ciated with neuroarthropathy of the foot and ankle. Brodsky and Rouse[6] classified neuroarthropathy based on location: disease in the midfoot (type 1), the hindfoot (type 2), the ankle (type 3a), and avulsion fracture of the calcaneus by the Achilles tendon (type 3b). Disease in multiple locations was classified as type 4, and disease in the forefoot was classified as type 5.

In 1998, Sammarco and Conti,[20] and Schon and colleagues[27] described similar radiographic classification systems of Charcot midfoot deformity associated with neu-roarthropathy. The Sammarco classification was presented with a series of 27 patients who had midfoot neuroarthropathy and were treated with surgical reduction and arthrodesis[20] (**Fig. 1**). Five patterns were identified: pattern 1—diastasis of the first and second metatarsals with fragmentation and collapse extending across the tarso-metatarsal joint; pattern 2—medial metatarsal-cuneiform destruction without diastasis of the first and second metatarsals; pattern 3—arthropathy at the navicular-medial cuneiform joint with fragmentation of the middle cuneiform and destruction across the lateral tarsometatarsal joints; pattern 4—arthropathy of the first metatarsal-medial cuneiform joint with diastasis between the first and second metatarsals and proximal and lateral extension into the intercuneiform joints ending at the calcaneocuboid joint; and pattern 5—perinavicular arthropathy with distal intertarsal extension.

Later that year, Schon and colleagues[27] published radiographic and clinical classifi-cation systems for midfoot neuropathic deformity (**Fig. 2**). The radiographic classifica-tion was developed after reviewing the weight-bearing radiographs of 131 neuroarthropathic feet. This classification is based on the anatomic area of involvement: type I—Lisfranc pattern; type II—naviculocuneiform pattern; type III—perinavicular pattern; and type IV—transverse tarsal (Chopart) pattern. These investigators also intro-duced a clinical classification system based on the degree of deformity seen on physical examination while weight bearing. In stage A, the midtarsus was above the metatarso-calcaneal plane. In stage B, the midtarsus was coplanar with this plane. In stage C, the midtarsus was below this plane (**Fig. 3**). In 2002, Schon and colleagues[28] published an interobserver reliability and reproducibility study to validate the proposed radiographic classification. Seventy-five orthopedists were tested, and the system was found to be reliable, with lower error rates among foot and ankle subspecialists and residents.

The degree of deformity is also important in classifying Charcot midfoot neuroarthr-opathy, because standardized angular measurements tend to normalize when the foot dislocates through the midfoot. In cases in which the midfoot has dislocated, the anteroposterior and lateral first tarsometatarsal angles tend to decrease with increasing deformity because following dislocation, the foot would develop a "bayonet" configuration, with the first metatarsal and talus becoming parallel.

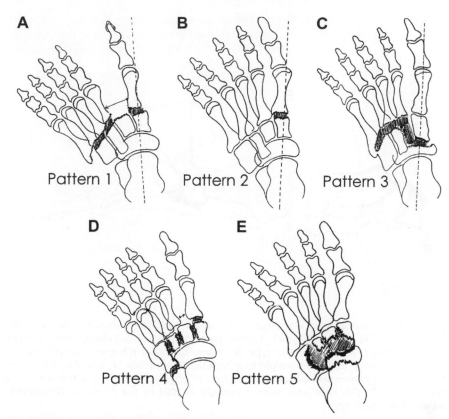

Fig. 1. Patterns of Charcot midfoot dislocation as described by Sammarco and Conti.[29] (*A*) Pattern 1: diastasis between the first and second metatarsals, with middle and lateral column dislocation/dissolution at the tarsometatarsal (TMT) joint. (*B*) Pattern 2: first TMT joint involvement only. (*C*) Pattern 3: medial column dislocation at the naviculocuneiform joint, with TMT joint dislocation of the middle and lateral columns. (*D*) Pattern 4: first TMT joint dislocation with first-second metatarsal diastasis, intercuneiform fragmentation, and extension to the calcaneocuboid joint. (*E*) Pattern 5: perinavicular arthropathy with distal intertarsal fragmentation and extension. (*From* Sammarco GJ, Conti SF. Surgical treatment of neuropathic foot deformity. Foot Ankle Int 1998;19:105; with permission. Copyright © 2009 by the American Orthopaedic Foot and Ankle Society.)

Sammarco and Conti[20] included a measurement of dorsal displacement to quantify the degree of midfoot deformity, and this measurement was better defined by Sammarco and colleagues[29] in a series of patients who underwent midfoot reconstruction for neuroarthropathic deformity. Dorsal displacement was measured on the lateral radiograph as the vertical distance between the axis of the talus and the axis of the first metatarsal at the level of the midfoot dislocation (**Fig. 4**). On the weight-bearing lateral radiograph, a line perpendicular to the floor was drawn at the apex of the deformity, the difference in height from the floor to the line was drawn down the central axis of the talus, and the central axis of the first metatarsal was measured. Schon and colleagues[28] classified the degree of deformity as type alpha or beta. A beta stage indicates more severe deformity and is assigned when one or more of the following criteria are met: (1) a dislocation is present, (2) the lateral first metatarsal angle is 30° or greater, (3) the lateral calcaneal-fifth metatarsal angle is 0° or greater, or (4)

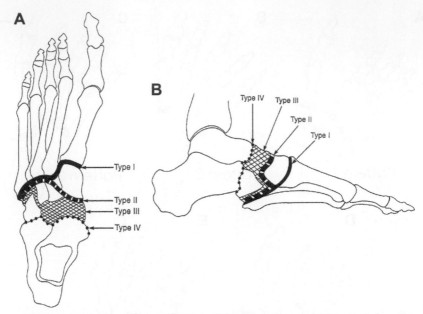

Fig. 2. Schon and colleague's[27] classification of diabetic midtarsus deformity is based on the anatomic area of involvement: type I—Lisfranc pattern; type II—naviculocuneiform pattern; type III—perinavicular pattern; and type IV—transverse tarsal (Chopart) pattern. (*A*) A/P weight bearing x-ray. (*B*) Lateral weight bearing x-ray. (*From* Schon LC, Weinfeld SB, Horton GA, et al. Radiographic and clinical classification of acquired midtarsus deformities. Foot Ankle Int 1998;19:397; with permission. Copyright © 2009 by the American Orthopaedic Foot and Ankle Society.)

the anteroposterior talar-first metatarsal angle is 35° or greater. Schon and colleagues[28] used standardized views with weight-bearing radiographs of the foot to determine the alpha-beta classification, using angular measurements described by Gould[30] and by Sangeorzan and colleagues.[31]

Sammarco and colleagues[29] recently used these classifications to evaluate the effectiveness of treatment in a series of patients treated with midfoot fusion and deformity correction for neuroarthropathy. In this series, patients who had Sammarco patterns 1 and 3 (Schon types 1 and 2) had better clinical results and fewer postsurgical complications. The high prevalence of the Schon beta designation and the significant amount of dorsal displacement in most patients indicated that the severity of deformity played a more important role in the decision for surgery than the anatomic pattern of involvement. Sammarco pattern 5 and Schon type 3 involve fragmentation of the navicular with involvement of the perinavicular joints, and required arthrodesis of the talonavicular joint in all cases and arthrodesis of the subtalar joint in two cases. Although successful results were eventually achieved, complications occurred in all seven of the Sammarco pattern 5/Schon type 3 deformities, with four patients suffering mechanical failure of the medial column fixation.

PREOPERATIVE MANAGEMENT

Preoperative assessment is of critical importance in achieving a successful clinical result. A thorough work-up for infection is necessary in many cases because the presence of osteomyelitis drastically changes the recommended treatment protocol. Many

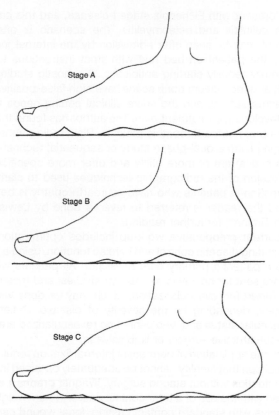

Fig. 3. Schon and colleague's[27] clinical stages of the degree of deformity are based on physical examination. In stage (A), the midtarsus is above the metatarsocalcaneal plane. In stage (B), the midtarsus is coplanar with this plane. In stage (C), the midtarsus is below this plane. (*From* Schon LC, Weinfeld SB, Horton GA, et al. Radiographic and clinical classification of acquired midtarsus deformities. Foot Ankle Int 1998;19:398; with permission. Copyright © 2009 by the American Orthopaedic Foot and Ankle Society.)

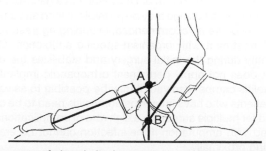

Fig. 4. The measurement of dorsal displacement in midfoot dislocation as described by Sammarco and colleagues.[29] The amount of dorsal displacement is the vertical distance measured between the midline of the lateral talar line at the level of dislocation (point B) and the midline of the lateral first metatarsal axis (point A) measured on weight-bearing radiographs. (*From* Sammarco VJ. Midtarsal arthrodesis in the treatment of Charcot midfoot arthropathy. J Bone Joint Surg Am 2009;91:80–91; with permission.)

Charcot patients present with Eichenolz stage I disease, and this can be difficult to differentiate from cellulitis and osteomyelitis. The scenario is often complicated because the patient may be seen after admission by the internal medicine service, which has placed the patient on bed rest with strict instructions to keep the foot elevated while simultaneously starting antibiotics. Diagnostic studies such as plain radiographs, MRI, and technetium bone scans have high false-positive rates for osteomyelitis in the acute setting, and the entire clinical setting needs to be evaluated carefully before developing a treatment plan. The author has found that MRI is of little utility in the work-up of neuroarthropathic patients. Plain radiographs combined with radionuclide imaging (with a dual-phase study or sequential technetium and labeled white blood cells scans) are of more utility and offer more specificity for infection. An in-depth discussion of the radiographic techniques used to clarify the presence or absence of infection in patients who have neuroarthropathy is beyond the scope of this article, and the reader is referred to reviews done by Lewis,[32] Lipman and colleagues,[33] and Timins[34] for further reading.

The author's current preoperative work-up includes optimization of all medical comorbidities, including diabetic control and cardiac function, using a team of medical specialists and the patient's primary care physician. All patients who do not have palpable pulses are sent for noninvasive vascular studies, and those who have poor vascularity are referred for revascularization, which may be done with endovascular or open techniques, depending on the severity of disease. Patients who do not have adequate vascular status and who cannot be revascularized are not considered candidates for reconstructive surgery or limb salvage.

Arthrodesis with the application of permanent internal fixation requires a sterile field. It is the author's opinion that sterility cannot be adequately obtained in the presence of ulcers or a deep infection without staged surgery. Wagner grades 1 and 2 ulcers can usually be resolved with the use of a total-contact cast and non–weight bearing. If the ulcers do not resolve with standard contact casting, local wound care, and medical/vascular optimization, then a higher suspicion of osteomyelitis should be present. Patients who are unable to resolve ulcers despite optimized medical treatment may not have adequate biologic resources to heal surgical wounds and arthrodesis procedures. These patients may be better served with primary amputation.

Cases in which neuroarthropathic foot deformity is combined with osteomyelitis represent a particularly difficult subset of patients. Patients in whom infection cannot be ruled out with standard imaging and radiographic criteria should undergo biopsy and are surgery planned accordingly. In patients who have neuropathic foot deformity combined with infection, limb salvage may be possible. If limb salvage is to be attempted, then a staged procedure is recommended, including aggressive debridement of infected bone and treatment with organism-specific antibiotics. Often, the author reduces the deformity during the initial surgery and stabilizes the extremity with an external fixator but does not apply permanent orthopaedic implants in this setting. When the osteomyelitis can be resolved, it may be possible to salvage the extremity with arthrodesis. Patients who have known osteomyelitis need to be counseled preoperatively of the need for multiple surgeries, a high rate of complications, and the potential need to proceed with amputation if the infection cannot be eradicated or if the infection is spreading proximally.

"SUPERCONSTRUCTS"

Neuropathic midfoot disease is inherently difficult to treat surgically. "Dissolution" of the bone in the area of fracture with resultant dislocation is one of the hallmarks of the disease process and is thought to be caused by sympathetic denervation and a resultant hyperemia. Bony dissolution, fragmentation, and osteoporosis increase the technical demands of midfoot reconstruction in neuropathic fractures. Earlier series reported recurrence of the deformity and nonunion as common sequelae of attempted arthrodesis. Standard fixation techniques using obliquely oriented lag screws are often inadequate due to the bony changes that accompany the Charcot process (**Fig. 5**). Poor bone quality, neuropathy, poor vascularity, and impaired nutrition of glycosylated tissue in diabetic patients all delay healing of the arthrodesis and contribute to complications. Patients are often overweight and inflexible and may find it difficult or impossible to comply with the non–weight bearing restrictions needed to achieve arthrodesis.

Evolving techniques have focused on increasing the stability of fixation primarily by extending fixation hardware proximally and distally into areas where the bone is not fragmented by the neuropathic process. Small-diameter crossed screws and pins are being replaced by larger, stronger fixation devices. Newer techniques do not depend on the poor bone in the area of dissolution for fixation but "bridge" this area by achieving fixation proximally and distally. Although this methodology sacrifices motion in otherwise normal joints, the stability of these constructs is dramatically improved.

The term *superconstruct* may be used to describe surgical techniques in which some normal principles of orthopaedic techniques are abandoned to improve stability and diminish the likelihood of failure of the procedure. A superconstruct is defined by four factors: (1) fusion is extended beyond the zone of injury to include joints that are not affected to improve fixation, (2) bone resection is performed to shorten the extremity to allow for adequate reduction of deformity without undue tension on the soft tissue envelope, (3) the strongest device is used that can be tolerated by the soft tissue envelope, and (4) the devices are applied in a position that maximizes mechanical function. Superconstructs are used in cases in which technical problems in achieving a successful surgical outcome are expected. Superconstructs are often performed in the settings of bone loss, dysvascular bone, major deformity correction, and severe osteoporosis, and in patients who have multiple medical comorbidities that make them high risk for poor surgical healing. These cases involve fusion of joints that are not involved in the area of pathology to improve the fixation of the construct.

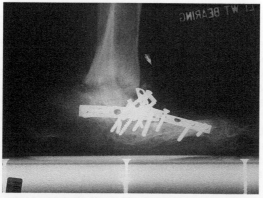

Fig. 5. Lateral radiograph of failed midfoot reconstruction done with crossed small-diameter screws and one-third tubular plates applied dorsally and medially. Note the recurrence of deformity and mechanical failure of multiple implants.

A superconstruct often uses orthopaedic implants that are stronger than those normally used to achieve arthrodesis, and those implants may be placed in a manner that optimizes their mechanical advantage despite technical difficulties in using these techniques. This article discusses three evolving superconstruct methods of achieving correction and fusion in patients who have neuroarthropathic foot disease: plantar plating, locked plating, and axial screw fixation. These techniques are new, with limited data from the literature available for review.

Plantar Plating Techniques

Although the application of plates for fixation of midfoot fusions is not new, plating has been a popular method of fixation of fusions in patients who have Charcot midfoot disease. Plating allows the fixation to span the area of Charcot dissolution into areas of better-quality bone. When the plates are extended into the metatarsals, fixation can be placed into cortical bone, which usually has better density than the midfoot bones. Plating can also be used to add compression to the fusion site. Due to anatomic considerations and technical ease of placement, dorsal and medial applications of plate constructs have been the most common. Despite extension of the fusion into uninvolved and better bone, however, plate fixation alone does not seem to significantly improve union rates in neuropathic feet. Schon recognized that application of plates in a plantar location offered multiple mechanical advantages, despite technical difficulties in applying the device in this location (Schon LC, MD, personal communication, 1998). Schon developed the concept of plantar plating to improve the strength of the construct, noting that the plantar location would improve the intraoperative ability to achieve correction and place the device under tension during weight bearing (Schon LC, MD, personal communication, 1998). In a simulated midfoot fusion model, Marks and colleagues[35] showed that application of the plates plantarly was biomechanically more stable than crossed screws in stiffness and in load to failure. A similar study comparing plantar plate fixation with screw fixation for metatarsal osteotomies yielded similar results.[36] The construct yields superior strength by placing the plate along the tension side of the fusion mass (**Fig. 6**). Schon and colleagues[21] reported successful results using this technique in 34 patients who had severe midfoot neuroarthropathic disease that had failed conservative and other surgical measures. The author has found plantar plating techniques to produce reliable arthrodesis of neuropathic midfoot dislocation.

Locked Plating

The use of locked plates, which were developed as fixed-angle devices for fixation of long-bone fractures, has expanded almost exponentially over the past few years. These devices create a fixed-angle device by rigidly attaching the screw to the plate. These devices have the advantage of significantly improving fixation in osteoporotic bone.[37,38] For Charcot midfoot disease, these devices have many desirable traits. The fixed-angle device overcomes some of the difficulties of applying the plate plantarly. In theory, the locked plate has equivalent fixation to the plantar construct, without necessitating the extensile plantar exposure needed for the latter. In cases in which the talonavicular joint must be crossed, the author has found it difficult to apply any plate plantarly due to the sustentaculum tali of the calcaneus. A medial or dorsal plate can achieve excellent fixation in the talar neck without necessitating fusion of the subtalar joint (**Fig. 7**). The author is unaware of any published clinical series of Charcot disease being treated with locked plates for fixation, although the technique was presented at the American Academy of Orthopaedic Surgeons Specialty Day (V. James Sammarco, MD, unpublished data, 2008).

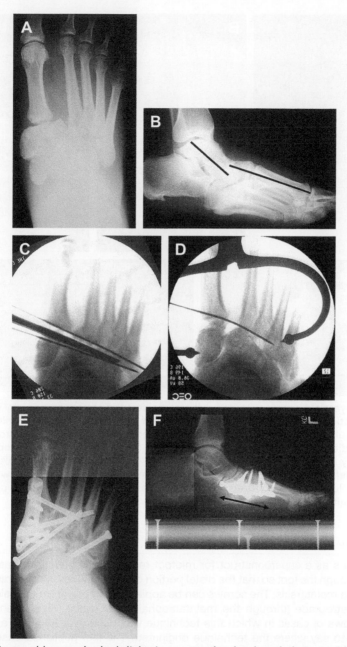

Fig. 6. A 36-year-old man who had diabetic neuropathy developed Charcot midfoot dislocation after a minor trauma and was treated with midfoot osteotomy and arthrodesis. (*A* and *B*) Preoperative radiographs. (*C* and *D*) Intraoperative fluoroscopy showing plantar medial resection of bone as described by Schon and colleagues.[21] (*E* and *F*) Two-year postoperative radiographs show solid fusion. Note that plantar plate is along tension side of fusion mass.

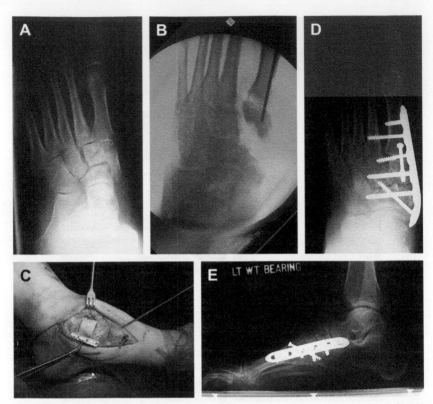

Fig. 7. A 48-year-old woman who had diabetes mellitus and sensory neuropathy developed an atraumatic dislocation of the medial column of her foot, with bony prominence and impending ulceration. (*A*) Preoperative anteroposterior radiograph shows Charcot dislocation of medial column at naviculocuneiform joint. (*B*) Intraoperative fluoroscopy demonstrates bony defect caused by dissolution of bone. (*C*) Allograft iliac crest graft is shaped to fit the defect. (*D* and *E*) Radiographs taken 18 months postoperatively show successful fusion with locking plate construct. The plate acts as a fixed-angle device and can be contoured to suit the anatomy.

Axial Screw Fixation

Axial screws as a superconstruct for midfoot reconstruction refers to passing long screws through the foot so that the distal portion of the screw lies in the intramedullary canal of the metatarsals. The screws can be applied antegrade (from the calcaneus or talus) or retrograde (through the metatarsophalangeal joints) (**Figs. 8** and **9**). The author knows of cases in which this technique was used over 20 years ago, and it is difficult to say where the technique originated. The first published case that the author is aware of was presented for reconstruction of a midfoot deformity in which a screw was passed from the calcaneus into the fourth metatarsal shaft.[39] Kann and colleagues[26] demonstrated that axial screw placement afforded better stability than an oblique screw in fusion of the calcaneocuboid joint.

The technique of applying multiple axial screws as fixation has several advantages. The first is that the placement and positioning of the screws aid in reduction of the deformity. Temporary fixation can be achieved with guide wires for cannulated screws, allowing the foot position and radiographs to be checked before application

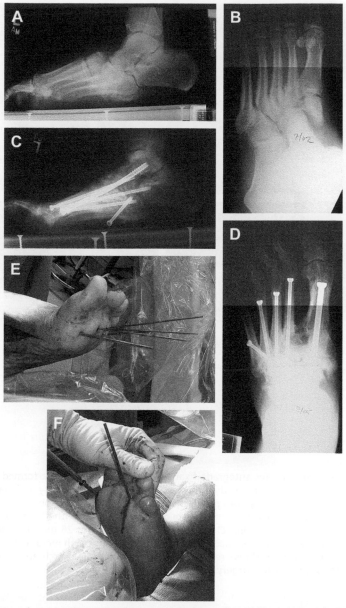

Fig. 8. This case demonstrates retrograde axial fixation of a midfoot fusion done for neuro-arthropathy in a 54-year-old man who had diabetes mellitus. (*A* and *B*) Preoperative radiographs show dislocation through the midfoot. (*C* and *D*) Radiographs taken 3 years following surgery show successful fusion and good maintenance of reduction. (*E* and *F*) Screw insertion technique. The deformity is reduced and final positioning is temporarily achieved by passing guide wires for cannulated screws through the metarsophalangeal joints. Final positioning is then checked fluoroscopically. The metatarsal shafts are reamed with cannulated drills so that they will accept larger-diameter screws without shattering. Screws are applied through the metarsophalangeal joints and countersunk to the level of the distal metaphyseal-diaphyseal junction.

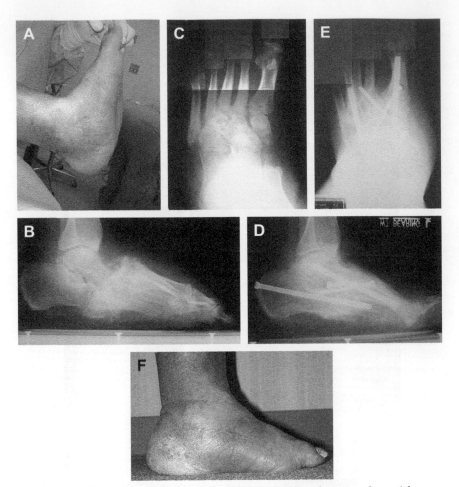

Fig. 9. This case demonstrates antegrade fixation of a midfoot fusion performed for neuro-arthropathy in a 37-year-old man who had severe peripheral neuropathy and diabetes mellitus. (*A*) Preoperative clinical photograph shows Schon stage C rocker-bottom deformity. (*B* and *C*) Preoperative radiographs showing midfoot dislocation with "bayoneting" of the forefoot on the hindfoot. (*D* and *E*). Postoperative radiographs 26 months after midfoot fusion using antegrade intramedullary screws in the first and fourth metatarsals. (*F*) Postoperative clinical photograph shows restoration of the longitudinal arch and a plantigrade foot more than 2 years after surgery.

of the final fixation devices. Compression of the arthrodesis sites is accomplished by simply tightening the screws. The intramedullary positioning of the screws eliminates stress risers in the cortical bone of the metatarsals that occur from transcortical screws created with plates or oblique screws. In addition, the fusion procedures can be done through more limited incisions without the extensive stripping of bone necessary for the application of long plates. The screw position is entirely intraosseous, which diminishes concern for exposed hardware in the event of a wound complication.

Sammarco and colleagues[29] recently published a series of patients who had neuro-arthropathic midfoot deformity treated with midfoot fusion using intramedullary screws for correction and fixation. Twenty-two patients were followed for an average 52 months (minimum 2 years' follow-up). The indications for surgery were recurrent ulcerations and gross instability that was not amenable to management with custom diabetic shoewear or a Charcot restraint orthotic walker. The patients had severe disease, and 20 of the 22 patients were classified as Schon type beta due to dislocation of the midfoot or severe angular deformity. Patients in whom the fusion crossed the talonavicular joint were at higher risk for complications and nonunion. At final follow-up, there were no amputations, and all patients were considered to have successful limb salvage.

SUMMARY

Management of Charcot deformity of the foot and ankle continues to challenge physicians. Medical comorbidity, peripheral neuropathy, vascular disease, and immune impairment cause severe problems for these patients and, when combined with neuroarthropathy, can lead to amputation. Progressive bony deformity and bone resorption, which may accompany neuroarthropathy, only increase the challenge of surgical treatment. These challenges have led physicians to develop superconstruct techniques whereby fusion is extended beyond the zone of injury to include joints that are not affected to improve fixation, bone resection is performed to shorten the extremity to allow for adequate reduction of deformity without undue tension on the soft tissue envelope, the strongest device is used that can be tolerated by the soft tissue envelope, and the devices are applied in a novel position that maximizes mechanical function. Large clinical series are lacking, but early reports of these new techniques are promising.

REFERENCES

1. Charcot J. Sur quelques arthropathies qai paraisant dependre d'une lesion du cervau on de la moelle epinere. Arch Physiol 1868;(1):161–78 [in French].
2. Jordan W. Neuritic manifestations in diabetes mellitus. Arch Intern Med 1936;57: 307–36.
3. Helm PA, Walker SC, Pullium G. Total contact casting in diabetic patients with neuropathic foot ulcerations. Arch Phys Mcd Rehabil 1984;65:691–3.
4. Walker SC, Helm PA, Pullium G. Total contact casting and chronic diabetic neuropathic foot ulcerations: healing rates by wound location. Arch Phys Med Rehabil 1987;68:217–21.
5. Walker SC, Helm PA, Pullium G. Total-contact casting, sandals, and insoles. Construction and applications in a total foot-care program. Clin Podiatr Med Surg 1995;12:63–73.
6. Brodsky JW, Rouse AM. Exostectomy for symptomatic bony prominences in diabetic Charcot feet. Clin Orthop Relat Res 1993;296:21–6.
7. Harrelson JM. The diabetic foot: Charcot arthropathy. Instr Course Lect 1993;42: 141–6.
8. Lesko P, Maurer RC. Talonavicular dislocations and midfoot arthropathy in neuropathic diabetic feet. Natural course and principles of treatment. Clin Orthop Relat Res 1989;240:226–31.
9. Leventen EO. Charcot foot—a technique for treatment of chronic plantar ulcer by saucerization and primary closure. Foot Ankle 1986;6:295–9.
10. Piaggesi A, Schipani E, Campi F, et al. Conservative surgical approach versus non-surgical management for diabetic neuropathic foot ulcers: a randomized trial. Diabet Med 1998;15:412–7.

11. Alvarez RG, Barbour TM, Perkins TD. Tibiocalcaneal arthrodesis for nonbrace-able neuropathic ankle deformity. Foot Ankle Int 1994;15:354–9.

12. Bono JV, Roger DJ, Jacobs RL. Surgical arthrodesis of the neuropathic foot. A salvage procedure. Clin Orthop 1993;296:14–20.

13. Campbell JT. Intra-articular neuropathic fracture of the calcaneal body treated by open reduction and subtalar arthrodesis. Foot Ankle Int 2001;22:440–4.

14. Cooper PS. Application of external fixators for management of Charcot defor-mities of the foot and ankle. Foot Ankle Clin 2002;7:207–54.

15. Early JS, Hansen ST. Surgical reconstruction of the diabetic foot: a salvage approach for midfoot collapse. Foot Ankle Int 1996;17:325–30.

16. Johnson JE. Surgical treatment for neuropathic arthropathy of the foot and ankle. Instr Course Lect 1999;48:269–77.

17. Myerson MS, Henderson MR, Saxby T, et al. Management of midfoot diabetic neuroarthropathy. Foot Ankle Int 1994;15:233–41.

18. Pakarinen TK, Laine HJ, Honkonen SE, et al. Charcot arthropathy of the dia-betic foot. Current concepts and review of 36 cases. Scand J Surg 2002;91: 195–201.

19. Papa J, Myerson M, Girard P. Salvage, with arthrodesis, in intractable diabetic neuropathic arthropathy of the foot and ankle. J Bone Joint Surg Am 1993;75: 1056–66.

20. Sammarco GJ, Conti SF. Surgical treatment of neuroarthropathic foot deformity. Foot Ankle Int 1998;19:102–9.

21. Schon LC, Easley ME, Weinfeld SB. Charcot neuroarthropathy of the foot and ankle. Clin Orthop 1998;116–31.

22. Schon LC, Marks RM. The management of neuroarthropathic fracture-disloca-tions in the diabetic patient. Orthop Clin North Am 1995;26:375–92.

23. Simon SR, Tejwani SG, Wilson DL, et al. Arthrodesis as an early alternative to nonoperative management of Charcot arthropathy of the diabetic foot. J Bone Joint Surg Am 2000;82:939–50.

24. Stone NC, Daniels TR. Midfoot and hindfoot arthrodeses in diabetic Charcot arthropathy. Can J Surg 2000;43:449–55.

25. Bohannon RW, Kelly CB. Accuracy of weightbearing at three target levels during bilateral upright stance in patients with neuropathic feet and control subjects. Percept Mot Skills 1991;72:19–24.

26. Kann JN, Parks BG, Schon LC. Biomechanical evaluation of two different screw positions for fusion of the calcaneocuboid joint. Foot Ankle Int 1999;20:33–6.

27. Schon LC, Weinfeld SB, Horton GA, et al. Radiographic and clinical classification of acquired midtarsus deformities. Foot Ankle Int 1998;19:394–404.

28. Schon LC, Easley ME, Cohen I, et al. The acquired midtarsus deformity classifi-cation system—interobserver reliability and intraobserver reproducibility. Foot Ankle Int 2002;23:30–6.

29. Sammarco VJ, Sammarco GJ, Walker EW Jr, et al. Midtarsal arthrodesis in the treatment of Charcot midfoot arthropathy. J Bone Joint Surg Am 2009;91:80–91.

30. Gould N. Graphing the adult foot and ankle. Foot Ankle 1982;2:213–9.

31. Sangeorzan BJ, Mosca V, Hansen ST Jr. Effect of calcaneal lengthening on rela-tionships among the hindfoot, midfoot, and forefoot. Foot Ankle 1993;14:136–41.

32. Lewis P. Scintigraphy in the foot and ankle. Foot Ankle Clin 2000;5:1–27.

33. Lipman BT, Collier BD, Carrera GF, et al. Detection of osteomyelitis in the neuro-pathic foot: nuclear medicine, MRI and conventional radiography. Clin Nucl Med 1998;23:77–82.

34. Timins ME. MR imaging of the foot and ankle. Foot Ankle Clin 2000;5:83–101, vi.

35. Marks RM, Parks BG, Schon LC. Midfoot fusion technique for neuroarthropathic feet: biomechanical analysis and rationale. Foot Ankle Int 1998;19:507–10.
36. Campbell JT, Schon LC, Parks BG, et al. Mechanical comparison of biplanar proximal closing wedge osteotomy with plantar plate fixation versus crescentic osteotomy with screw fixation for the correction of metatarsus primus varus. Foot Ankle Int 1998;19:293–9.
37. Haidukewych GJ, Ricci W. Locked plating in orthopaedic trauma: a clinical update. J Am Acad Orthop Surg 2008;16:347–55.
38. Tejwani NC, Wolinsky P. The changing face of orthopaedic trauma: locked plating and minimally invasive techniques. Instr Course Lect 2008;57:3–9.
39. Sammarco GJ. Chapter 11: diabetic arthropathy. In: Sammarco GJ, editor. The foot in diabetes. Philadelphia: Lea and Febiger; 1991. p. 153–72.

Skewfoot

Sebastién Hagmann, MD, Thomas Dreher, MD,
Wolfram Wenz, MD*

KEYWORDS

• Skewfoot • Metatarsus adductus • Z-shaped foot
• Serpentine foot • McHale procedure

Skewfoot is a rare deformity characterized by combined forefoot adduction and hindfoot valgus (**Fig. 1**). Currently, the literature dealing with this deformity remains sparse. To the authors' knowledge, there have been fewer than 20 original articles directly treating the topic. A few cases have also been discussed in connection with other, more common deformities.

TERMINOLOGY

An initial description of the deformity was given by Henke in 1863.[1] Seventy years later, in 1933, a first review of the literature and a description of 14 cases was reported by Peabody and Muro,[2] which concluded that the combination of hindfoot valgus and forefoot adduction was different from metatarsus adductus due to its resistance to the effects of therapy. They therefore labeled the deformity "congenital metatarsus varus" to differentiate it from the more common metatarsus adductus. Only in 1949 was the term *skewfoot* coined by McCormick and Blount,[3] who used it as a generic term for deformities such as metatarsus varus, metatarsus adductus, metatarsus adductovarus, and metatarsus adductocavovarus. Other investigators have had a share in adding to the terminologic confusion by proposing the terms metatarsus adductus, serpentine metatarsus adductus, Z-shaped foot, and S-shaped foot.[4]

In this regard, when speaking of a foot deformity that matches the criteria for forefoot adduction and hindfoot valgus, the authors recommend using terms that clearly discriminate this deformity from metatarsus adductus, such as skewfoot, serpentine foot, or Z-shaped foot.

INCIDENCE AND ETIOLOGY

The incidence of skewfoot is unknown but may be underestimated due to the common misdiagnosis of metatarsus adductus. Most investigators have concluded that it is

Division of Pediatric Orthopaedics and Foot Surgery, Orthopaedic Department, University of Heidelberg, Schlierbacher Landstrasse 200a, Heidelberg 69118, Germany
* Corresponding author.
E-mail address: wolfram.wenz@ok.uni-heidelberg.de (W. Wenz).

Foot Ankle Clin N Am 14 (2009) 409–434
doi:10.1016/j.fcl.2009.06.003
1083-7515/09/$ – see front matter © 2009 Elsevier Inc. All rights reserved.

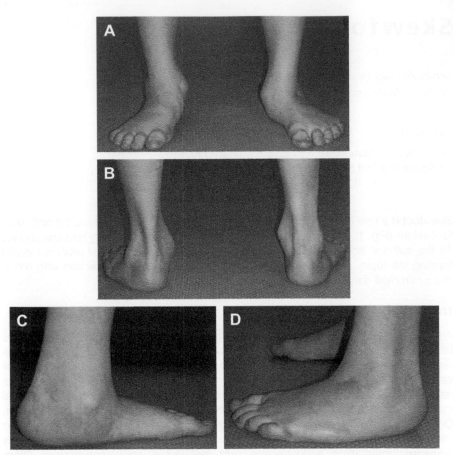

Fig.1. Clinical presentation of skewfoot. (*A*) Front view shows bilateral forefoot adduction. (*B*) Rear view shows bilateral hindfoot valgus. (*C*) The medial aspect of the foot shows pes planus deformity. (*D*) The lateral aspect of the foot is C-shaped, as in metatarsus adductus.

a rare but therapeutically challenging deformity. Kite[5] reported only 12 serpentine feet in 2818 feet that had metatarsus adductus. He found a strong hereditary influence in these patients and a high resistance to conservative treatment.

Due to the higher incidence of metatarsus adductus, its etiology is much better understood than the etiology of skewfoot. Several causal correlations for the development of metatarsus adductus have been proposed and seem to also be applicable to skewfoot. Because metatarsus adductus is present at birth in most cases but is not observed in preterm infants,[6] a role of intrauterine position in the development of the deformity has been suggested. Some investigators, therefore, assume that intrauterine position might play a role in congenital idiopathic skewfoot.[7]

Moreover, muscle imbalance may play a role in the development of metatarsus adductus. A predominance of tibialis anterior, tibialis posterior, and adductor hallucis muscles vis-à-vis the peroneal muscles has been discussed. Muscle imbalance due to anatomic variations of tendon insertion has been proposed in the case of skewfoot. Peabody and Muro[2] reported a variation in the insertion of the tibialis anterior tendon, comparable to Tönnis[7] finding a more distally inserting tibialis anterior tendon. By contrast, Napiontek[8] reported an intraoperative observation that the tibialis anterior tendon lies more proximally and passes through the medial aspect of the medial cuneiform-navicular joint. In some cases, he observed a severe deformation of the medial cuneiform. This finding corresponds with Mosca's[9] observation of the distal tibialis anterior lying in a groove on the concave medial cortex of a varied medial cuneiform. By contrast, MRI examinations of 16 children (27 feet) who had skewfoot did not show any abnormalities in the course of the tendons.[10] The significance of all these anatomic findings, however, remains functionally unclear. So far, there has not been a convincing hypothesis on the etiology of skewfoot. It is for this reason that skewfoot is often discussed in the context of metatarsus adductus, whereas in other cases, it is dealt with in the context of flatfoot.

Some early investigators who focused on skewfoot presumed that this distinct deformity developed from other foot deformities in the course of therapy; however, MRI examinations of untreated children who had not begun walking showed the typical aspects of the deformity, refuting the assumption that all of the deformity develops with treatment or on weight bearing.[10] Apart from these congenital cases, clinical experience has shown that the deformity can be seen in the context of neurogenic or systemic disorders and as a result of nonoperative or operative foot-deformity treatment. Variations in the severity of the deformity and of its response to therapy make it necessary to discern one skewfoot from the other.

CLASSIFICATION

Napiontek,[8] therefore, proposed a classification scheme to distinguish four clinical types of the deformity:

Congenital idiopathic skewfoot
Congenital skewfoot associated with syndromes or systemic disorders
Neurogenic
Iatrogenic skewfoot

Congenital idiopathic skewfoot is the most controversially discussed. To this day, there is uncertainty concerning the natural evolution of the deformity. Some investigators have assumed that the deformity resolves with time—as it appears to do so with most metatarsus adductus cases—and have therefore been critical of therapeutic intervention.[11] The literature and clinical practice to date, together with MRI findings, however, attest to the existence of congenital skewfoot.

Skewfoot has been reported to occur in diastrophic dwarfism, osteogenesis imperfecta, and other syndromes such as Larsen's syndrome and Proteus syndrome.[12–15] It also seems to appear in relation to certain connective tissue diseases such as Ehlers-Danlos syndrome (Fig. 2). Skewfoot in these populations is often found to be rigid and difficult to treat.

All major neurogenic disorders in children (eg, cerebral palsy or myelodysplasia) are thought capable of developing skewfoot deformity. To the authors' knowledge, due to the muscular imbalance leading or adding to the deformity, therapeutic management is a considerable challenge in these cases. Progression of the deformity is most often faster than in idiopathic cases, sometimes unfolding into extreme cases (Fig. 3).

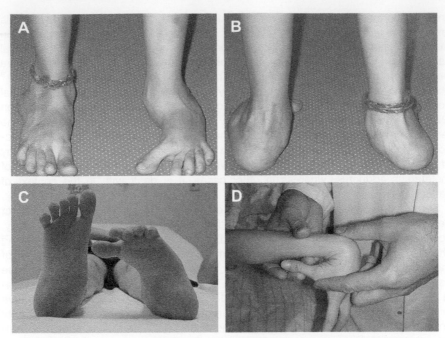

Fig. 2. Skewfoot in a girl who has an unclear connective tissue disorder. (*A*) Front view. (*B*) Rear view. (*C*) View from below. (*D*) Joint hypermobility is present in all joints.

Iatrogenic skewfoot is most likely a result of nonoperative clubfoot or metatarsus adductus treatment (**Fig. 4**). In cases of resistant forefoot adduction in clubfoot, apparent correction can be produced through the midfoot, with lateral translation of the navicular and cuboid at Chopart's joint. Hindfoot overcorrection in clubfeet (eg, in plaster cast therapy) can cause valgus deformity. As a result of the opposite deformities, feet can appear normal, and therapeutic success can be mistakenly assumed.

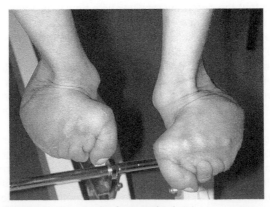

Fig. 3. Severe skewfoot in a patient who has cerebral palsy.

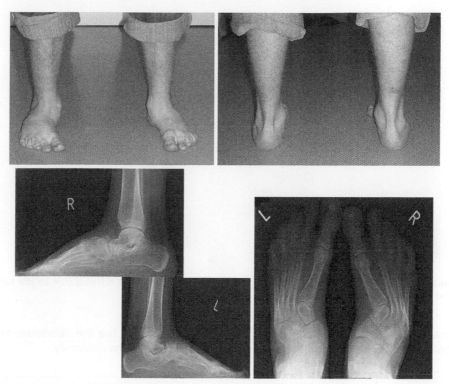

Fig. 4. Iatrogenic bilateral skewfoot after conservative clubfoot treatment. Due to their opposite directions, the deformities tend to cancel each other out clinically. Radiographs reveal the amount of midfoot malalignment, especially on the right side.

CLINICAL EXAMINATION

Diagnosis of skewfoot is based on clinical and radiologic confirmation of forefoot adduction and hindfoot valgus. It must be distinguished from simple metatarsus adductus, equinovarus, and flatfoot deformity. Skewfoot should also be suspected when infants do not respond to treatment for metatarsus adductus.[16] The deformity should be assessed by examination in a standing position and by inspection of the plantar and dorsal aspects of the foot. The appraisal of tibial torsion is crucial for differential diagnosis and for potential therapeutic management. In children younger than 1 year, hindfoot valgus may easily be overlooked due to the hindfoot fat and the more apparent forefoot adduction. Therefore, the deformity can be misdiagnosed as metatarsus adductus (**Fig. 5**). Unlike for metatarsus adductus,[17] the "V-finger test" is not helpful in most cases because the antipodal components may mask the actual severity of the deformity. In fact, because of the neutralizing directions of the deformity, in some cases, the foot can appear normal in standing position. In this regard, skewfoot can be compared to scoliosis.

During examination, the mobility of joints should be assessed. Stiffness of the deformity is considered to be a sign of rather unfavorable prognosis regarding spontaneous restitution. Clinical photographs should be taken in standing and reclined positions to document progression or therapeutic success. Alternatively, a simple method of documentation consists of taking photocopies of the feet with simulated weight

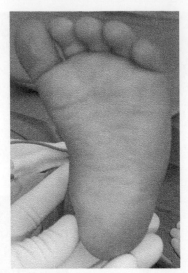

Fig. 5. Metatarsus adductus. Assessment of hindfoot valgus may be difficult due to the fat pad in children under 1 year of age.

bearing, as in metatarsus adductus.[18] This method, however, has the disadvantage that information is lost concerning the nonplantar aspects of the deformity.

RADIOLOGIC EXAMINATIONS

Simple metatarsus adductus usually does not need to be objectified by radiologic examinations. In contrast, when suspecting skewfoot, anteroposterior and lateral radiographs with weight bearing are recommended. Radiographs of the ankle joint should be taken to rule out accompanying anatomic variations that may affect treatment. Lloyd-Roberts and Clark[19] reported two cases of skewfoot with ball-and-socket ankle joints that were unfavorable to treatment. In situations in which is it not possible to obtain weight-bearing radiographs due to the age of the patient or disability, radiographs should be taken with simulated weight bearing, as proposed by Berg.[20] Such radiographs can be achieved with x-ray–permeable slats. Anteroposterior radiographs reveal forefoot adduction, midfoot abduction, and hindfoot valgus, creating the serpentine aspect of the deformity (**Fig. 6**). Lateral radiographs reveal hindfoot valgus and pathology of the midfoot. It should be noted that proper radiographic technique is crucial for analysis of the radiograph. Improper technique should be ruled out before analysis according to fixed radiographic criteria in children.[21,22]

The degree of forefoot adduction is determined by analysis of the talo–first metatarsal angle (**Fig. 7**). This angle best describes forefoot adduction, because deviation of the first metatarsal is greater than that of the lateral metatarsals.[22] There is consensus on defining forefoot adduction as medial deviation of the first metatarsal compared to the talar axis. In this case, the talo–first metatarsal angle should be documented with a negative value.

Measurement of the talocalcaneal angle in anteroposterior and lateral radiographs reveals the severity of hindfoot valgus (see **Fig. 7**). Evaluation can be difficult depending on the radiographic aspect of the talus and calcaneus, especially in young infants. Measurements should be compared to age-related normal values because angles differ in relation to the age of the patient.[23]

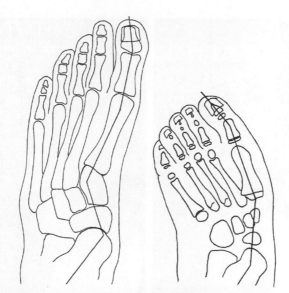

Fig. 6. Radiologic aspect of skewfoot (*left image*). The changing directions of the deformity have led to such terms as serpentine foot, S-shaped foot, or Z-shaped foot. Forefoot adduction and hindfoot valgus tend to cancel each other out clinically. (*Right side*) In contrast, pes planus. (*From* Döderlein L, Wenz W, Schneider U. Der Knickplattfuß. Berlin/Heidelberg/New York: Springer; 2002. p. 134; with permission.)

In anteroposterior and lateral radiographs, the navicular is often found to be laterally abducted and dorsiflexed from the talar head. Lateral subluxation of the navicular on the head of the talus is a cardinal radiographic sign of skewfoot. Documentation of lateral talonavicular subluxation is dependent on navicular ossification, which is often delayed in patients who have skewfoot.[22] In contrast to the navicular, the medial cuneiform is medially shifted and plantarflexed.

It is important to note that in skewfoot, the opposite direction of the deformities can cancel each other out. This situation can be reflected in a normal talo–first metatarsal angle measurement. Mosca[9] reported 8 of 10 skewfoot patients as having normal talo–first metatarsal angles despite clinically severe skewfoot.

MRI can provide further information in some cases. Compared with radiography, MRI has the advantage of being able to show the cartilaginous and ossified portions of the developing bones. A disadvantage, however, is that weight bearing or simulated weight bearing is not possible, and therefore meaningful angles cannot be measured.[10]

In the authors' opinion, MRI and CT scanning can be useful in severe deformities to provide information about osseous and cartilage conditions. In most cases, however, it is not part of the standard pretherapeutic assessment. Most of the information needed for diagnosis and treatment can be taken from standard radiographs even if ossification is not advanced.[10]

There have been some attempts to establish a radiographic classification for skewfoot. In 1986, Berg[20] proposed a classification for metatarsus adductus and skewfoot based on anteroposterior and lateral radiographs. Four types of deformity were distinguished: simple metatarsus adductus, complex metatarsus adductus, simple skewfoot, and complex skewfoot. The classification was based on a scheme first evaluating malalignment of the midfoot, as characterized by lateralization of the

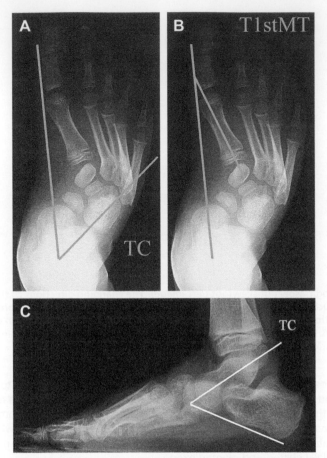

Fig. 7. Important angles used to define the degree of the deformity. (*A*) Talocalcaneal (TC) angle in the anteroposterior plane, defined as the angle of the direct axis of the talus and the direct axis of the calcaneus. (*B*) Talo–first metatarsal (T1stMT) angle, defined as the angle between direct axis of the talus and direct axis through the first metatarsal bone. (*C*) TC angle in the sagittal plane.

cuboid in respect to the calcaneal line. Malalignment of the middle part of the foot is defined as a "complex" deformity. Metatarsus adductus and skewfoot are both characterized by medial angulation of the talus–first metatarsal line. Skewfoot, in Berg's classification, is additionally characterized by a talocalcaneal angle greater than 35° on the anteroposterior and 45° on the lateral radiograph.

Criticism of this classification was mostly due to the high interobserver disagreement and intraobserver inconsistency, as revealed by Cook and colleagues.[24] These investigators could not detect a correlation between the classification and the time needed for successful cast treatment. Berg's classification, however, remains a helpful tool in objectifying the severity of the deformity. Berg[20] showed that the duration of conservative treatment increased from simple metatarsus adductus to complex skewfoot. It should nevertheless be said that the classification is not able to guide therapeutic decisions.

Another attempt at classification was made by Bensahel and Desgrippes,[25] on the basis of changes in the first metatarsal and talar angle on anteroposterior radiographs.

In metatarsus adductus, the longitudinal axes of the first metatarsal and talus cross just before the proximal end of the first metatarsal, whereas in first-degree skewfoot, the axes cross at the first metatarsal diaphysis. In second-degree skewfoot, they cross distally from the second phalanx of the great toe, whereas third-degree skewfoot is characterized by parallelism of both axes. As for Berg's classification, the main criticism is that no therapeutic implication has been shown for the Bensahel and Degrippes' distinction of the deformities.

Therefore, the decision of when and how to treat remains an assignment for the orthopedic surgeon.

THERAPY

Therapy in skewfoot deformity is controversial. One problem is that the natural history of skewfoot is unknown. Some investigators believe that some of the deformities might correct spontaneously with age, as is observed in metatarsus adductus[11] or flatfoot.[26] To date, however, there is no long-term follow-up study of untreated versus treated skewfoot that reveals the amount of spontaneous correction in the deformity.

Theoretically, the following measures of therapy can be taken into consideration:[7-9,14-16]

Manipulation
Serial casting
Orthoses
Surgical management

Some investigators believe that asymptomatic skewfoot in older children needs no treatment. There is no clear definition of where to draw an age line of when to treat and when not to treat. As for metatarsus adductus, the earlier the treatment begins, the more effectively the deformity can be treated by conservative means. In infants, manipulation and serial casting may be beneficial, but the most important question remains when to treat the deformity at all.

It is important to evaluate clinical response to any treatment initiated. When there is no response to treatment or when there is progression of the deformity, other means should be taken into consideration. The authors believe that in the treatment of skewfoot, stretching exercises and activity modification—methods often favored by parents—are not able to change the deformity, especially in older children.

There is no general consensus about therapeutic escalation. Due to the unknown natural history of skewfoot and due to the great differences regarding severity depending on the etiology, up to now, decisions about therapy remain the duty of the orthopedic surgeon.

It must be said that skewfoot associated with syndromes and neurologic disorders should be approached differently than idiopathic skewfoot or iatrogenic skewfoot. Therapeutic consideration, therefore, is not only a question of age but also of etiology and related to the probability of progression.

It goes without saying that symptomatic deformities should be treated. In children, symptoms due to foot deformities are infrequent. The main difficulty, therefore, remains detection of the deformities that need treatment because of the progression of symptoms or the presumption of their development. Most investigators agree that skewfoot associated with neurologic disorders and associated with syndromes should be treated earlier and more aggressively than idiopathic skewfoot.[8] The same approach might be applied to iatrogenic deformities, especially when there is clinical and radiologic progression.

It is justifiable to simply observe very mild deformities in very young children. Berg[20] showed that some cases of skewfoot in his study did not need treatment; however, intensive follow-up is important to detect progression.

Unlike for metatarsus adductus, the authors recommend manipulation of the feet only in young children who have mild deformities. Parents can be instructed in the technique of manipulation under supervision. Again, it is crucial to have intensive follow-up to check the efficacy of treatment. When there is a progression of the deformity, other measures should be employed.

In mild deformities without rigid components, serial plaster casting is an effective method. The main risk of serial casting is the progression of hindfoot valgus due to an improper technique. For that reason, the hindfoot should be retained in mild varus.

Berg[20] corrected adduction of the forefoot with the use of serial casts in metatarsus adductus and in skewfoot. He reported excellent results, with only 1 of 124 feet having residual forefoot adduction. In all other feet, a normal talo–first metatarsal angle was restored. As mentioned earlier, restoration of the talo–first metatarsal angle was also the case for untreated feet. The duration of casting that was necessary for correction was significantly longer in the patients who had skewfoot. Forty-one of the patients developed flatfoot deformity, which was mostly seen in feet that had been treated with a Denis-Brown bar for internal tibial torsion.

In more severe cases and in feet that show a progression of the deformity, especially under conservative treatment, operative procedures should be considered.

In younger children, consideration should be given to soft-tissue releases without (or with only limited) bony procedures, particularly if the deformity is flexible. Asirvatham and Stevens[27] treated 12 feet that had metatarsus adductus and 17 feet that had skewfoot by medial capsulotomy and adductor hallucis lengthening. In these young patients (average age, 3.6 years), good results could be seen at a mean follow-up of 3.6 years, with all of the feet having an improved talo–first metatarsal angle. Postoperative casting is thought to be essential to conserve correction.

Opening wedge osteotomy of the medial cuneiform has proved to be an adequate therapy for correction of forefoot varus.[28] On the other hand, calcaneal lengthening, as in the Evans osteotomy, has shown to be an excellent tool in flatfoot correction.

Mosca,[29] therefore, proposed a technique for skewfoot correction consisting of a calcaneal lengthening osteotomy modified from the technique of Evans, a Fowler medial cuneiform opening wedge osteotomy, and lengthening of the Achilles tendon. He reported satisfactory results in 9 of 10 feet that were thus treated.

Advantages of medial cuneiform opening wedge osteotomy, in comparison to first tarsometatarsal arthrodesis, for example, is that first-ray mobility is preserved and the amount of correction can easily be varied. In some cases, overgrowth of the medial cuneiform is observed due to division of the ossification center by the osteotomy.[30]

The question of whether to address hindfoot deformity is controversial. In 1990, Jawish and colleagues[31] reported on 55 cases of skewfoot in 31 children. Therapy was conservative in 15 feet and surgical in 29 feet, with 50% bad results. The investigators insisted on conservative treatment before the age of 1 year, with surgical treatment applied in case of failure of conservative treatment or in older children. Of interest, surgical correction of hindfoot together with correction of varus deformity led to transverse tarsal instability. The investigators therefore suggested correcting forefoot deformity by medial cuneiform and cuboid osteotomy without changing hindfoot anatomy. They shared the belief of Lloyd-Roberts and Clark[19] that the hindfoot deformity is flexible and might ameliorate with the course of time. The hindfoot was also not addressed by Coleman,[32] who proposed medial cuneiform opening wedge osteotomy and plantar fasciotomy.

In the authors' opinion, combining lateral column lengthening with a medial cunei-form osteotomy is not only esthetically important. Biomechanical cadaver studies of flatfoot have shown that medial cuneiform osteotomy reduces pressure under the lateral forefoot when a calcaneal lengthening is performed.[33] This principle should also be valid for skewfoot correction. The authors therefore recommend treating the hindfoot together with the forefoot. Treating only one deformity might cause deterio-ration of the other (**Figs. 8** and **9**).

In severe cases, medial cuneiform osteotomy might not be sufficient for correction of forefoot varus, but in general, this can be determined preoperatively. Because the amount of correction by medial cuneiform osteotomy does not usually exceed 10° in anteroposterior radiographs and 20° in lateral radiographs,[28] additional cuboid closing wedge osteotomy can be performed (McHale procedure, see later discussion). In more severe cases, closing wedge calcaneocuboid arthrodesis might be needed to provide sufficient correction.

Achilles tendon lengthening is an important step in the case of a contracted Achilles tendon, which is often present in severe flatfoot and skewfoot. According to the amount of contracture, other techniques such as intramuscular lengthening might be sufficient.

Other possibilities of correction depend on the age of the patient and the rigidity of the deformity. Kendrick and Herndon[34] proposed subtalar fusion or triple arthrodesis with forefoot correction, which might be applied when correction cannot be achieved by conserving the joints. In these cases, forefoot correction might only be achieved by multiple metatarsal osteotomies, or again, tarsometatarsal fusion (**Figs. 10** and **11**).

Fixateur externe therapy has not been reported in larger series but can offer excel-lent possibilities for correction to the experienced surgeon (**Fig. 12**).

It should be mentioned that there is no standard procedure for skewfoot. Most often, adequate treatment relies on the experience of the surgeon and can include a combination of osseous and nonosseous procedures (**Fig. 13**).

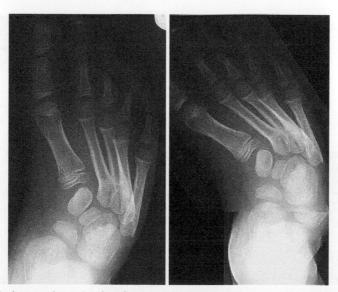

Fig. 8. Surgical procedures in skewfoot cause several problems. Correction of hindfoot deformity alone might deteriorate forefoot adduction.

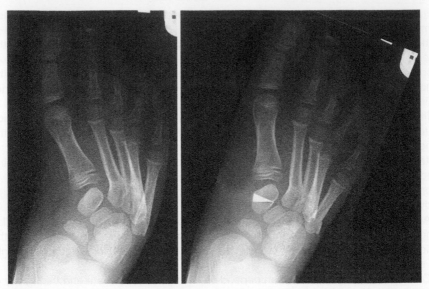

Fig. 9. Surgical procedures in skewfoot cause several problems. Correction of forefoot defor-mity alone can cause pes planus deformity.

SURGICAL TECHNIQUES
Anesthesia and Positioning

In general, all of the operations described in this section can be performed under spinal or general anesthesia, depending on the age of the patient. The authors place the patient in a supine position, with the possibility of sterile draping of the ipsilateral

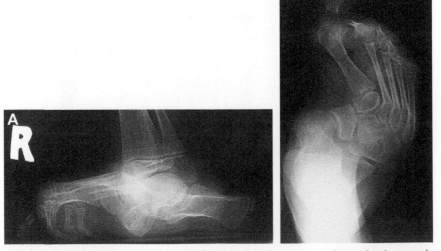

Fig. 10. (A, B) Preoperative radiographs of severe skewfoot in a patient who has cerebral palsy. The clinical aspect is shown in **Fig. 3.**

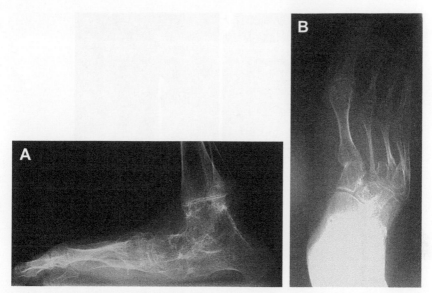

Fig. 11. (*A*, *B*) Postoperative radiographs of severe skewfoot in a patient who has cerebral palsy. Triple arthrodesis and tarsometatarsal fusion was required for correction.

or, in the case of prior surgery, the contralateral anterior iliac crest. A thigh tourniquet is utilized.

Sterile cover is extended to the knee to allow gastrocnemius recession if necessary and to allow intraoperative assessment of tibial torsion.

Evans Osteotomy

This procedure is a variation of the technique described by Evans.[35] The sinus tarsi is identified, followed by a straight lateral incision following the skin lines, centered over the anterior process of the calcaneus and extending to the calcaneocuboid joint. The subcutaneous tissue is dissected, and the sural and superficial branches of the peroneal nerve are identified and protected by applying loops (**Fig. 14**). The peroneus

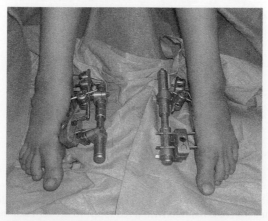

Fig. 12. Treatment of skewfoot by fixateur externe.

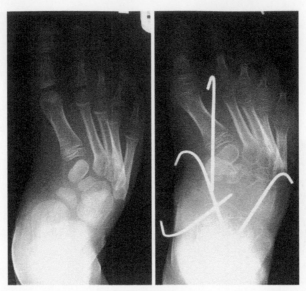

Fig. 13. Pre- (*left*) and postoperative (*right*) radiographs of skewfoot treated by medial cuneiform osteotomy and open soft-tissue release of the midfoot. Although midfoot alignment is restored, forefoot adduction remains.

longus and brevis tendons are retracted plantarward; the extensor digitorum brevis is elevated from the dorsal surface of the calcaneus and shifted distally. The calcaneocuboid joint is identified. One Hohmann retractor is placed on the plantar aspect; another is placed on the dorsal aspect of the anterior process of the calcaneus, anterior to the sinus tarsi (**Fig. 15**). The periosteum is then incised in the direction of the planned osteotomy, approximately 1.5 cm proximal to the calcaneocuboid joint. The osteotomy is then marked with a chisel before making the first part of the osteotomy with an oscillating saw under permanent cooling. The saw blade is inserted into the calcaneus while conserving the medial, dorsal, and plantar cortex (**Fig. 16**). The

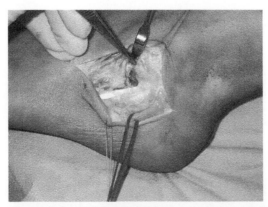

Fig. 14. Evans osteotomy. The sinus tarsi and the peroneal tendons are identified. The sural branch of the peroneal nerve is marked with a red loop. To prevent skin necrosis, the retraction is facilitated with two sutures.

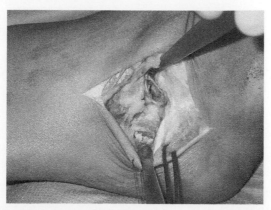

Fig. 15. Evans ostetomy. Two Hohmann retractors circumvent the anterior process of the calcaneus, approximately 1.5 cm proximal from the calcanocuboid joint.

saw blade is left in place and a Kirschner (K)-wire is placed from the cuboid through the distal fragment of the osteotomy to prevent dorsal deviation when completing the osteotomy (**Fig. 17**). The saw blade can be used as a target for the K-wire to provide sufficient fixation of the distal fragment. The osteotomy is then finished without sawing the medial cortex of the calcaneus, which is broken with the help of a chisel (**Fig. 18**). The osteotomy is then sufficiently mobilized, and two Steinmann pins are placed proximal and distal to the osteotomy. A K-wire distractor is installed and the osteotomy is spread until designated correction is reached (**Fig. 19**). Intraoperative radiographs are taken to assess the amount of correction needed. The size of the graft needed for correction is planned. A trapezoid-shaped graft is then taken from the iliac crest (**Fig. 20**). Depending on age and physical constitution, bi- or tricortical grafts are at the surgeon's disposal. The graft is then inserted (**Fig. 21**). Typically, correction remains stable after removal of the K-wire distractor. Although it may not be needed[29,36] due to primary stability, the authors fix the graft by advancing the previously installed K-wire through the graft and the proximal calcaneal fragment. Due to cost-effectiveness and handling, the authors prefer fixation by K-wires. With

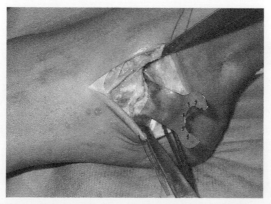

Fig. 16. Evans osteotomy. The saw blade is inserted without affecting the medial, dorsal, or plantar cortical shell of the calcaneus. It serves as a target for the K-wire (see **Fig. 17**).

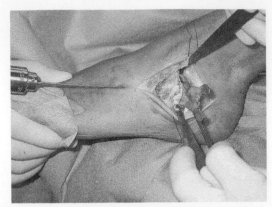

Fig. 17. Evans osteotomy. A K-wire is inserted through the cuboid for fixation of the distal fragment of the calcaneus, which prevents dorsal deviation when finishing the osteotomy.

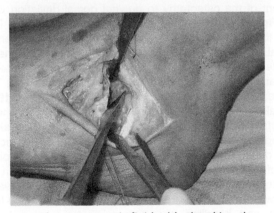

Fig. 18. Evans osteotomy. The osteotomy is finished by breaking the medial cortex of the calcaneus with a chisel.

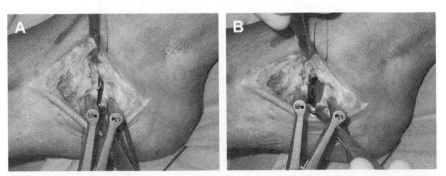

Fig. 19. (*A, B*) Evans osteotomy. A K-wire distractor helps to determine the amount of correction needed to reduce hindfoot valgus.

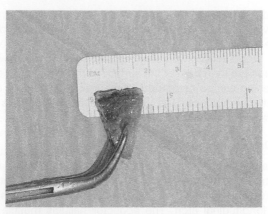

Fig. 20. Evans osteotomy. A trapezoid-shaped graft is taken from the iliac crest after determining the size of the osteotomy.

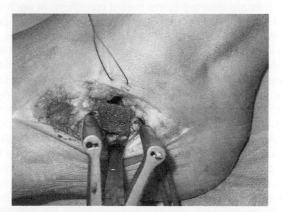

Fig. 21. Evans osteotomy. The graft is in place. Typically, correction remains stable after removal of the distractor.

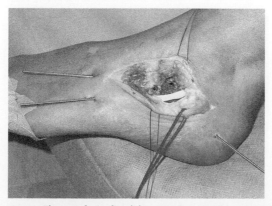

Fig. 22. Evans osteotomy. The graft is fixed by crossing K-wires. Depending on primary stability, two to four K-wires are inserted.

appropriate wound management, the risk of infection is minimized, and no implants remain after removal. Screw and plate fixation are also adequate, depending on the preferences of the surgeon. Another K-wire is inserted in the opposite direction for rotational stability. Depending on primary stability, two to four K-wires are inserted (**Fig. 22**). The K-wires are then bent at the surface of the skin for retrieval in the outpatient clinic. An opening wedge osteotomy of the medial cuneiform can then be performed to correct the forefoot. The postoperative treatment is detailed in the section "Postoperative treatment."

Opening Wedge Osteotomy of the Medial Cuneiform

This procedure is a variation of the technique described by Fowler and colleagues.[37] A skin incision is made on the medial aspect of the foot after detection of the medial cuneiform and the adjacent joints (**Fig. 23**). The direction of the incision should follow the shape of the longitudinal arch. The abductor hallucis muscle is exposed and divided from the medial border of the foot. The tibialis anterior tendon is retracted (**Fig. 24**); in some cases, it has to be detached on the level of the medial cuneiform. The capsules of cuneonavicular and cuneometatarsal first joints are identified (**Fig. 25**). Two K-wires are inserted in the medial cuneiform at each side of the level of osteotomy and cut at a length of approximately 3 cm. Under protection of the surrounding soft tissues, an osteotomy of the medial cuneiform is performed with an oscillating saw with permanent cooling or with a chisel (**Fig. 26**). A K-wire distractor is installed using the two K-wires inserted previously. Alternatively, the distraction can be done by the assistant (**Fig. 27**). The amount of correction needed is performed. In severe cases, the osteotomy may have to be shifted more laterally, including the middle cuneiform. The osteotomy is fixed in the desired position. A measurement is taken to match a fitting graft. The graft is then inserted into the osteotomy space (**Figs. 28** and **29**). Again, and especially in very young patients, the authors prefer fixation by K-wires. Screw or plate fixation, as mentioned earlier, might be an adequate means of fixation, depending on the size of the medial cuneiform. Two K-wires are inserted, with one wire passing from the first metatarsal through the medial cuneiform, the graft, and the navicular (**Fig. 30**). The other K-wire should pass through the navicular, medial cuneiform, the graft, and the first metatarsal for rotational stability. Depending on the amount of plantar flexion of the great toe, flexor hallucis longus elongation might be necessary. If the tibialis anterior tendon had to be detached, it needs to be reattached by leaving one half of the tendon at a length of 3 to 4 cm

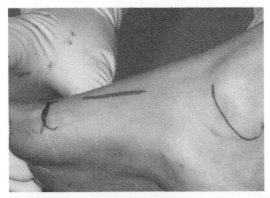

Fig. 23. Osteotomy of the medial cuneiform. Skin incision is made over the medial cuneiform and follows the direction of the longitudinal arch.

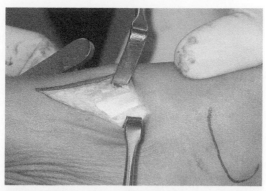

Fig. 24. Osteotomy of the medial cuneiform. After dissection of the subcutaneous tissue, the tibialis anterior tendon is identified.

attached to the bone. In this case, side-to-side tendon suture is sufficient. Wound closure is performed. The postoperative treatment is detailed in the section "Postoperative treatment."

Closing Wedge Osteotomy of the Cuboid and Opening Wedge Osteotomy of the Medial Cuneiform

This procedure is a variation of the technique described by McHale and Lenhart.[38] As mentioned earlier, the possibility of addressing forefoot adduction with a single opening wedge osteotomy of the medial cuneiform is limited. It might therefore be necessary to combine this procedure with a closing wedge osteotomy of the cuboid. A desired correction of more than 10° in the anteroposterior and 20° in the sagittal plane, in general, requires osteotomy of both bones. In this case, the procedure is started with the cuboid. Therefore, the skin is incised over 4 to 5 cm in the direction of the cuboid (**Fig. 31**). In the case of prior Evans osteotomy, the incision has to be extended distally. The subcuteaneous tissue is divided, and the extensor digitorum brevis muscle, the peroneus brevis tendon, and the distal branch of the sural nerve are identified (**Fig. 32**). The calcaneocuboid and tarsometatarsal joints are identified with the help of hollow needles (**Fig. 33**). In difficult cases, positioning should be

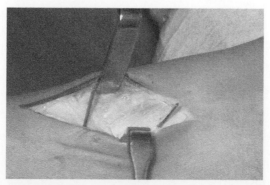

Fig. 25. Osteotomy of the medial cuneiform. The cuneometatarsal and cuneonavicular joints are identified with the help of hollow needles or thin K-wires. In difficult cases, intraoperative radiographs confirm proper localization.

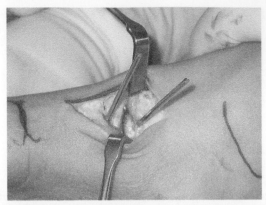

Fig. 26. Osteotomy of the medial cuneiform. The osteotomy has been made and two K-wires have been inserted on both sides of the osteotomy.

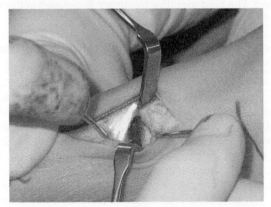

Fig. 27. Osteotomy of the medial cuneiform. The osteotomy is spread with a K-wire distractor or with the help of an assistant. The size of the graft needed is determined.

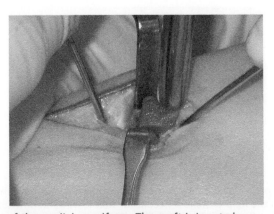

Fig. 28. Osteotomy of the medial cuneiform. The graft is inserted.

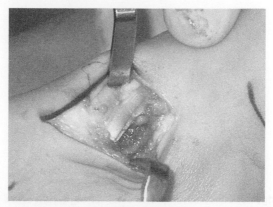

Fig. 29. Osteotomy of the medial cuneiform. The graft is in place. The tibialis anterior tendon covers the site of the osteotomy.

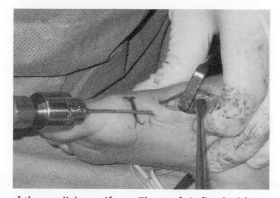

Fig. 30. Osteotomy of the medial cuneiform. The graft is fixed with two crossing K-wires.

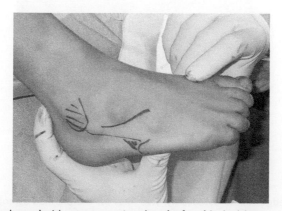

Fig. 31. Closing wedge cuboid osteotomy. Landmarks for skin incision.

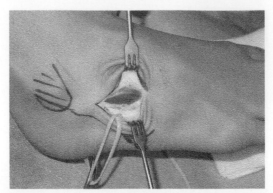

Fig. 32. Closing wedge cuboid osteotomy. The extensor digitorum brevis muscle, the peroneal tendons, and the distal branch of the sural nerve (*yellow loop*) are identified.

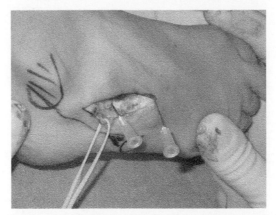

Fig. 33. Closing wedge cuboid osteotomy. Identification of calcaneocuboid and tarsometatarsal joints.

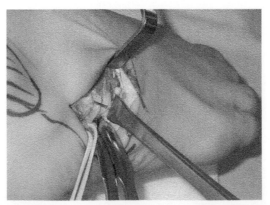

Fig. 34. Closing wedge cuboid osteotomy. Two lines for the planned osteotomy are marked with a chisel.

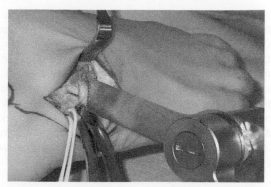

Fig. 35. Closing wedge cuboid osteotomy. A trapezoid-shaped osteotomy is made; the medial cuboid cortex is conserved.

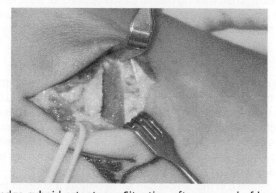

Fig. 36. Closing wedge cuboid osteotomy. Situation after removal of bone.

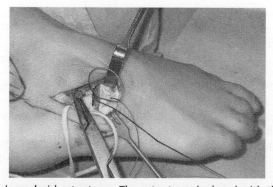

Fig. 37. Closing wedge cuboid osteotomy. The osteotomy is closed with the help of a transosseous absorbable suture.

assessed with the help of intraoperative radiographs. Two Hohmann retractors are placed at the plantar aspect of the cuboid. The dorsal aspect of the cuboid is exposed with a small Langenbeck clamp. The osteotomy is planned by making two grooves for the basis of the triangle with a chisel (**Fig. 34**). A laterally based triangle is then removed from the cuboid with an oscillating saw while cooling to prevent heat necrosis of the bone (**Figs. 35** and **36**). The medial cuboid cortex is conserved. The osteotomy is then closed with the help of an absorbable transosseus suture (**Fig. 37**). In older patients and when the surfaces of the osteotomy do not adapt sufficiently with the suture alone, two additional crossing K-wires or crossing screws can be inserted. Also, a small plate might be used for fixation. Subsequently, the medial cuneiform is addressed as mentioned earlier.

POSTOPERATIVE TREATMENT

Depending on the age of the patient, below- or above-knee plaster casts are applied. Depending on age and physical constitution, plaster casts remain for 4 to 6 weeks with absolute proscription of weight bearing. Plaster casts are changed every 2 weeks. After 4 to 6 weeks, radiographs are taken. The K-wires are then removed in the outpatient clinic and a below-knee walking plaster cast is applied for another 6 weeks. Weight bearing should be increased constantly, with full weight bearing around the 12th postoperative week in older patients and the eighth postoperative week in younger children.

SUMMARY

Skewfoot is a rare deformity and therefore might not present to an orthopedic surgeon not specialized in the correction of foot deformities. Skewfoot should be considered in the case of resistance to treatment measures when dealing with the more common metatarsus adductus. When diagnosed, therapy should be conducted by an orthopedic surgeon specialized in the correction of complex foot deformities. There is no consent about how and when to treat this deformity because its natural history is unknown. Numerous surgical procedures have been proposed.

The techniques detailed in this article can serve only as a support in the selection of an adequate therapy. The more complicated and severe the presenting deformity—as it often is in the case in noncongenital skewfoot—the more the surgeon will have to rely on his or her experience and intuition.

REFERENCES

1. Henke W. Handbuch der Anatomie und Mechanik der Gelenke [Handbook of anatomy and mechanics of the joints]. Leipzig, Heidelberg: C.F.Winter'sche Verlagsbuchhandlung; 1863 [in German].
2. Peabody CW, Muro F. Congenital metatarsus varus. J Bone Joint Surg 1933;15: 171–89.
3. McCormick DW, Blount WR. Metatarsus adductovarus. 'Skewfoot'. J Ann Med Assoc 1949;141:449–53.
4. Kite JH. Congenital metatarsus varus. Report of 300 cases. J Bone Joint Surg Am 1950;32:500–6.
5. Kite JH. Congenital metatarsus varus. J Bone Joint Surg Am 1967;49:388–97.
6. Katz K, Naor N, Merlob P, et al. Rotational deformities of the tibia and foot in preterm infants. J Pediatr Orthop 1990;10:483–5.
7. Tönnis D. [Skewfoot]. Orthopäde 1986;15:174–83 [in German].
8. Napiontek M. Skewfoot. J Pediatr Orthop 2002;22:130–3.

9. Mosca VS. Flexible flatfoot and skewfoot. J Bone Joint Surg Am 1995;77:1937–45.
10. Hubbard AM, Davidson RS, Meyer JS, et al. Magnetic resonance imaging of skewfoot. J Bone Joint Surg Am 1996;78:389–97.
11. Farsetti P, Weinstein SL, Ponseti IV. The long-term functional and radiographic outcomes of untreated and non-operatively treated metatarsus adductus. J Bone Joint Surg Am 1994;76:257–65.
12. Ryoppy S, Poussa M, Merikanto J, et al. Foot deformities in diastrophic dysplasia. J Bone Joint Surg Br 1992;74:441–4.
13. Mirzayan R, Cepkinian V, Yu J, et al. Skewfoot in patients with osteogenesis imperfecta. Foot Ankle Int 2000;2:768–71.
14. Napiontek M, Józwiak M. [Skewfoot—etiology, clinical appearance, management]. Chir Narzadow Ruchu Ortop Pol 1994;54:461–70 [in Polish].
15. Napiontek M, Józwiak M. Congenital skewfoot: clinical and radiographic appearance, management with emphasizing of surgical treatment. In: Epeldegui T, editor. Flatfoot and Forefoot Deformities. Madrid: A. Madrid Vincente: Ediciones; 1995. p. 296–304 [in Spanish].
16. Greene WB. Metatarsus adductus and skewfoot. Instr Course Lect 1994;43: 161–77.
17. Gore AI, Spencer JP. The newborn foot. Am Fam Physician 2004;69(4):865–72.
18. Smith JT, Bleck EE, Gamble JG, et al. Simple method of documenting metatarsus adductus. J Pediatr Orthop 1991;11(5):679–80.
19. Lloyd-Roberts GC, Clark RC. Ball and socket ankle joint in metatarsus adductus varus (S-shaped or serpentine foot). J Bone Joint Surg Br 1973;55:193–6.
20. Berg EE. A reappraisal of metatarsus adductus and skewfoot. J Bone Joint Surg Am 1986;68:1185–96.
21. Simons GW. A standardized method for the radiographic evaluation of clubfeet. Clin Orthop 1978;135:107–18.
22. Katz MA, Davidson RS, Chan PSH, et al. Plain radiographic evaluation of the pediatric foot and its deformities. UPOJ 1997;10:30–9.
23. Vanderwilde R, Staheli LT, Chew DE, et al. Measurements on radiographs of the foot in normal infants and children. J Bone Joint Surg Am 1988;70(3):407–15.
24. Cook DA, Breed AL, Cook T, et al. Observer variability in the radiographic measurement and classification of metatarsus adductus. J Pediatr Orthop 1992;12:86–9.
25. Bensahel H, Desgrippes Y. Metatarsus varus and skewfoot. In: Epeldegui T, editor. Flatfoot and Forefoot Deformities. Madrid: A. Madrid Vincente: Ediciones; 1995. p. 285–8 [in Spanish].
26. Staheli LT, Chew DE, Corbett M. The longitudinal arch. A survey of eight hundred and eighty-two feet in normal children and adults. J Bone Joint Surg Am 1987;69:426–8.
27. Asirvatham R, Stevens PM. Idiopathic forefoot-adduction deformity: medial capsulotomy and abductor hallucis lengthening for resistant and severe deformities. Pediatr Orthop 1997;17:496–500.
28. Hirose CB, Johnson JE. Plantarflexion opening wedge medial cuneiform osteotomy for correction of fixed forefoot varus associated with flatfoot deformity. Foot Ankle Int 2004;25:568–74.
29. Mosca VS. Calcaneal lengthening for valgus deformity of the hindfoot. Results in children who had severe, symptomatic flatfoot and skewfoot. J Bone Joint Surg Am 1995;77:500–12.
30. Napiontek M, Kotwicki T, Tomaszewski M. Opening wedge osteotomy of the medial cuneiform before age 4 years in the treatment of forefoot adduction. J Pediatr Orthop 2003;23:65–9.

31. Jawish R, Rigault P, Padovani JP, et al. The Z-shaped or serpentine foot in children and adolescents. Chir Pediatr 1990;31:314–21.
32. Coleman S. Complex foot deformities in children. Philadelphia: Lea and Febiger; 1983.
33. Benthien RA, Parks BG, Guyton GP, et al. Lateral column calcaneal lengthening, flexor digitorum longus transfer, and opening wedge medial cuneiform osteotomy for flexible flatfoot: a biomechanical study. Foot Ankle Int 2007;28:70–7.
34. Kendrick RF, Sharma NK, Hassler WL, et al. Tarsometatarsal mobilization for resistant adduction of the fore part of the foot. A follow-up study. J Bone and Joint Surg 1970;57A:61–70.
35. Evans D. Calcaneo-valgus deformity. J Bone Joint Surg Br 1975;57:270–8.
36. Hintermann B, Valderrabano V, Kundert HP. Lateral column lengthening by calcaneal osteotomy combined with soft tissue reconstruction for treatment of severe posterior tibial tendon dysfunction. Technique and preliminary results. Orthopäde 1999;28:760–9.
37. Fowler SB, Brooks AL, Parrish TF. The cavo-varus foot. J Bone Joint Surg Am 1959;41:757–61.
38. McHale KA, Lenhart MK. Treatment of residual clubfoot deformity—the "bean-shaped" foot—by opening wedge medial cuneiform osteotomy and closing wedge cuboid osteotomy. Clinical review and cadaver correlations. J Pediatr Orthop 1991;11:374–81.

Recurrent Clubfoot—Approach and Treatment with External Fixation

Ricardo Cardenuto Ferreira, MD[a],*, MarcoTúlio Costa, MD[b]

KEYWORDS

- Clubfoot • Treatment • Recurrent deformity • External fixator
- Osteotomy

The current treatment of congenital clubfoot in the newborn is nonsurgical. Although the majority of patients achieve satisfactory deformity correction with weekly serial manipulations and casting during the first 6 weeks of life, some feet cannot be adequately corrected with conservative treatment. The more rigid the initial deformity, the more likely surgical treatment is required. Corrective surgery for idiopathic clubfoot in children up to 1 year of age usually presents satisfactory results.[1,2] In approximately 20% of these patients, however, additional corrective surgery may be necessary because of recurrence of the deformity.

The treatment of recurrent clubfoot is challenging even for experienced surgeons. This deformity has a tendency to recur even after several corrective surgeries. Additional surgeries focused exclusively on the soft tissue may lead to greater joint stiffness. The tridimensional aspects of clubfoot deformity and the severe joint stiffness with retraction of soft tissues significantly limit the use of conventional corrective methods, such as osteotomies, triple arthrodesis, or talectomy. These surgical procedures are technically challenging due to the multiplanar and stiff deformities found in the clubfoot. A limitation of the corrective capacity of surgery is the typical shortened medial column of the foot associated with a tense neurovascular bundle.[3,4] When aggressive corrections of all the deformities are attempted in a single surgical procedure there is a great risk for damage to the neurovascular bundle, which usually is surrounded by and adhered to scar tissue (**Fig. 1**). Therefore, one-step surgical corrections are considered high risk. Another significant limitation to the use of tarsal osteotomies and conventional arthrodesis to treat recurrent clubfoot is the significant

[a] Division of Foot and Ankle, Department of Orthopaedics, Santa Casa School of Medicine and Hospitals, Rua Barata Ribeiro 380, sexto andar, São Paulo – SP, CEP 01308-000, Brazil
[b] Division of Foot and Ankle, Department of Orthopaedics, Santa Casa School of Medicine and Hospitals, Rua Dr. Cesário Motta Junior 112, São Paulo – SP, CEP 01222-000, Brazil
* Corresponding author.
E-mail address: ceckley@unisys.com.br (R.C. Ferreira).

Foot Ankle Clin N Am 14 (2009) 435–445
doi:10.1016/j.fcl.2009.03.009
1083-7515/09/$ – see front matter © 2009 Elsevier Inc. All rights reserved.

foot.theclinics.com

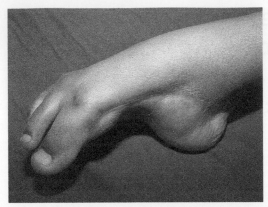

Fig.1. Lateral view of the right foot of an 11-year-old boy before treatment. Note the severe equinocavus deformities and the extensive scar formation in the medial side of the foot and ankle.

technical complexity, secondary to the tridimensional aspects of the deformity. The need to perform bone wedge resections leads to additional shortening of the foot.[5–17] Potential risks to the soft tissues include extensive skin necrosis, secondary infection, neurovascular compromise, and ischemia,[9,10] all of which may lead to amputation.

In the past decade the use of circular external fixators has become a treatment option for recurrent clubfeet. This treatment is based on the distraction-osteogenesis principles described by Ilizarov and colleagues.[13] The progressive distraction offered by the external fixator allows simultaneous correction of all components of the clubfoot deformity.[10,13] During the course of correction, a gradual lengthening of the blood vessels, nerves, muscles, connective tissues, and skin occurs, reducing the risks for neurovascular damage, skin necrosis, and secondary infection.[3,12] The Ilizarov method is safe and minimally invasive, requiring minimal or no bone resection.[6–8,10,12,18,19] Use of this method also offers more predictable and satisfactory results.[3,5–17] Another advantage of the Ilizarov external fixator over conventional methods is preservation of foot size or lengthening of a baseline shortened foot. Osteotomies of the midfoot or hindfoot should be performed during the distraction process in feet that have undergone previous arthrodesis. When such osteotomies are performed, the treatment period is prolonged and the device must be kept in place until bone consolidation is complete.[3]

One of the challenges associated with the treatment of foot deformities involves the frame setting of the Ilizarov circular external fixator. The device used for correction of clubfoot involves a significant number of connections and adjustments at different levels. This complexity creates difficulties for patients and for physicians during the course of treatment. The correction of the deformities themselves is challenging due to the complexity of variables involved. These factors significantly increase the learning curve of the method.[6,7] The use of a standard setting simplifies the method, allows better control of the course of correction, and reduces the learning curve of the method for surgeons in training.[6–8] The significant difference in the standard setting of the circular external fixator is the reduction in the number of hinges that require adjustments. In this simplified setting, the supination deformity is assessed only after the other deformities have been corrected. The previous distraction of soft tissue surrounding the joints and the midfoot osteotomy (in selected cases) makes correction of this remaining deformity less cumbersome.

INDICATIONS FOR TREATMENT

The main indication for the treatment of recurrent clubfoot with circular external fixation involves patients who present with a severely deformed foot with a stiff midfoot and hindfoot. Patients who have recurrent clubfoot typically present with extensive scarring of the skin that is deeply adhered to the posterior-medial neurovascular bundle of the foot. The predominant deformities are equinovarus and equinocavus greater than 30°, preventing patients from bearing weight on their heels and from wearing conventional shoes (**Fig. 2**). These anatomic characteristics are considered high risk for compromise to the neurovascular bundle and skin necrosis with a one-strike surgery.

SURGICAL TECHNIQUE

Correction of recurrent deformity may be performed using a simplified standard setting of the Ilizarov modular circular external fixator (**Fig. 3**) through gradual and progressive distraction of the soft tissues (joint, capsules, ligaments, tendons, and skin). A limited surgical approach is used with minor soft tissue dissection. Only two or three small incisions are necessary: one plantar of approximately 2.0 cm for plantar fasciotomy, one posterior of approximately 0.5 cm for percutaneous tenotomy of the Achilles tendon, and one medial of approximately 1.0 cm for posterior tibial tenotomy (**Fig. 4**). Ankylosis or malunion of a previous arthrodesis of the midfoot obligates a surgeon to perform a transverse midtarsal osteotomy. This procedure is performed through a single longitudinal dorsal or lateral approach (**Fig. 5**).

The simplified standard setting of the Ilizarov device[6,7,18] uses two parallel rings fixed perpendicular to the axis of the tibia by four crossed wires (1.5 or 1.8 mm in diameter), two for each ring, with a 110-N tension applied to the wires. The calcaneus is fixed with two crossed olive wires (1.5 or 1.8 mm in diameter) locked to a half-ring positioned parallel to the longitudinal axis of this bone. The wires are tensioned at 90-N. A 5-mm–diameter Schantz pin is introduced from the posterior region of the calcaneus tuberosity and directed along the axis of the calcaneus to enhance the

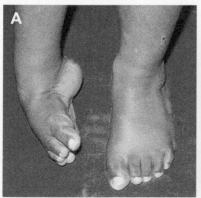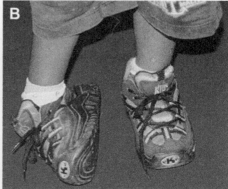

Fig. 2. Anterior view of the right foot of a 5-year-old boy who had an equinocavovarus deformity: (*A*) barefoot and (*B*) with shoe wear.

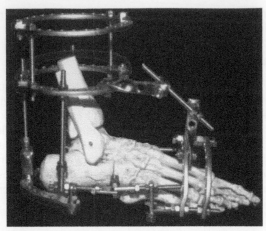

Fig. 3. Standard setting of the modular circular external fixator used to correct the deformities of recurrent clubfoot.

stability of the frame setting. Two olive wires (1.5 or 1.8 mm in diameter) are passed through the metatarsal bones to allow fixation of the forefoot; these wires are placed parallel to each other and fixed to a half-ring tensioned at 90-N. The two forefoot half-rings are positioned parallel to each other in the frontal plane and perpendicular to the axis of the forefoot. The rings and the half-rings are connected to each other using two threaded rods and hinges positioned so as to allow independent movement of the forefoot, midfoot, and hindfoot. No connection rods are placed between the tibial and the forefoot frames during this initial procedure (**Fig. 6**). Only after complete and gradual correction of the equinus, varus, cavus, and adduction deformities are achieved is attention paid to the supination deformity. Acute correction of the supination deformity is performed under general anesthesia (usually 12 weeks after the beginning of correction) followed by the placement of an anterior rod for stabilization.

POSTOPERATIVE CARE AND MANAGEMENT

Correction of the deformities starts 3 days after the placement of the Ilizarov device, in a gradual and progressive manner. Patients may remain in the hospital during most of the corrective period; this allows close monitoring of the neurovascular status. This

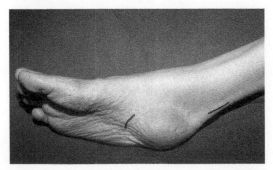

Fig. 4. Ink marks showing the site and size of incisions for plantar fasciotomy and Achilles tenotomy before placement of the modular circular external fixator.

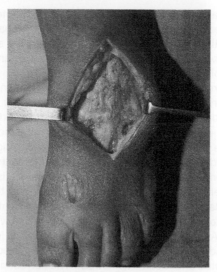

Fig. 5. Dorsolongitudinal approach used for transversal midtarsal osteotomy in recurrent clubfoot presenting previous malunited arthrodesis.

also facilitates daily physical therapy to prevent clawing of the toes, preserve knee mobility, and aid in early walking. In compliant patients who have access to outpatient physical therapy, inpatient hospital stay is not required. The speed of correction is based on a patient's capacity to withstand the pain caused by the distraction and on the circulatory, neurologic, and skin status. Progressive correction is achieved by two or three daily adjustments of the device. The hindfoot is corrected by lengthening the two posterior rods connecting the rings on the tibia to the half-ring on the calcaneus. The medial rod is lengthened faster than the lateral rod for simultaneous correction of the equinus and varus deformities. The adduction and cavus deformities of the midfoot and forefoot are corrected by lengthening the rods between the calcaneus and the forefoot. The medial rod is lengthened faster than the lateral rod to correct the adduction.

As discussed previously, the supination deformity is the last one to be corrected. Under general anesthesia, the connecting rods between the hindfoot setting

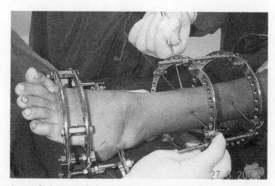

Fig. 6. Standard setting of the modular circular external fixator used to correct the deformities of recurrent clubfoot.

(connected to the calcaneus) and the forefoot setting (connected to the metatarsals) are temporarily removed. The foot is placed in mild hyperpronation of approximately 10° before the connecting rods are replaced. To enhance the stability of the setting, the final step of the procedure involves the placement of an anterior rod connecting the distal ring of the tibial frame to the forefoot.

The total time for correction is approximately 10 weeks (varying from 8 to 14 weeks), depending on the severity and stiffness of the deformities. After this corrective period, patients are discharged from the hospital (if inpatient) and the device is kept in place, with no further adjustments, for an additional 4 weeks, to achieve stabilization of the correction. Patients are allowed to bear weight on the foot using a customized rocker bottom sandal attached to the foot and the external fixator with self-adhesive straps. When midfoot osteotomies are made necessary, the device is kept in place for an additional approximately 8 weeks to ensure consolidation of the regenerated bone. After removal of the device under general anesthesia, patients are kept in a short leg-walking cast for another 4 to 6 weeks and encouraged to walk bearing full weight on the operated limb. After this period, an ankle-foot orthosis is used for 6 months.

There is no gold standard evaluation system to establish objective clinical results for the treatment of neglected and recurrent clubfoot. The correction of severe foot deformities associated with recurrent clubfoot significantly improves cosmetics and the potential to achieve a plantigrade functional foot capable of adapting to normal shoes, which ultimately improves patient quality of life and gait ability.[7,17]

Clinical criteria were established by Ferreira and colleagues[7] for the treatment of neglected clubfoot using the Ilizarov external fixator. Five criteria were analyzed: a painless foot and ankle, capacity to walk on a plantigrade foot, capacity to wear conventional shoes, absence of significant recurrence of the original deformity after a follow-up period of at least 2 years, and patient satisfaction with the final appearance of the foot. When all the criteria are met, the result is considered good; when only one of the criteria is not met, the result is considered fair; and when two or more of the criteria are not met, the result is considered poor. Based on these criteria, the results obtained by the authors and colleagues[18] with the treatment of 35 severely deformed and stiff recurrent clubfeet using a simplified standard setting of the Ilizarov external fixator in patients who had a mean age of 14 years (ranging from 4 to 31) were good in 27 feet (77%), fair in five feet (14%), and poor in three feet (9%) after a mean follow-up of 56 months (**Figs. 7** and **8**).

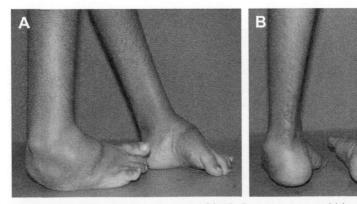

Fig. 7. Lateral (*A*) and posterior (*B*) views of both feet in a 7-year-old boy showing severe deformities before correction with the modular circular external fixator.

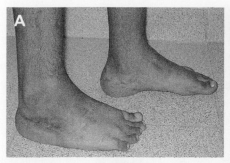
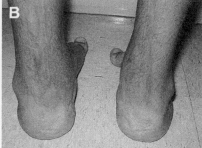

Fig. 8. Postcorrective aspect of the same boy depicted in **Fig. 7** (33- and 36-month follow-up for right and left foot, respectively). Note the plantigrade aspect of both feet in the lateral (*A*) and posterior views (*B*).

COMPLICATIONS

Complications associated with this method of treatment involve limited skin pin-tract infection to some extent in virtually every patient during the course of treatment, clawing of the toes (**Fig. 9**), and limited ischemia on the posterior-medial aspect of the foot and ankle. Local dressing and systemic antibiotics for a short period of time usually control the infections. Skin ischemia is treated by reducing the speed of correction. To avoid clawing of the toes, assisted physical therapy is recommended along with the use of a small orthosis made of leather and elastic bands. If the clawing of the toes persists despite conservative treatment, percutaneous tenotomy of the flexor tendon at the metatarsal-phalangeal groove followed by temporary fixation with intramedullary Kirschner wires during a 4-week period can satisfactorily correct the deformity (**Fig. 10**). Other unusual complications are subluxation or complete dislocation of the metatarsophalangeal joint of the hallux (**Fig. 11**), treated with periarticular soft tissue release, joint realignment, and temporary transarticular Kirschner wire fixation. In patients who have an immature skeleton, epiphysiolysis of the distal tibia eventually can occur during the period of joint distraction (**Fig. 12**). This complication has been observed by several investigators[2,7,17,20,21] but apparently does not require special attention or additional interventions, as spontaneous remodeling of the bone occurs during the course of the treatment with no apparent sequelae.[18] It is the authors' belief

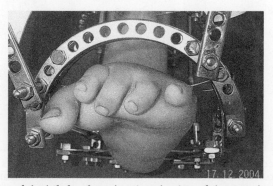

Fig. 9. Frontal aspect of the left forefoot showing clawing of the toes developed during the treatment of recurrent clubfoot with the modular external fixator.

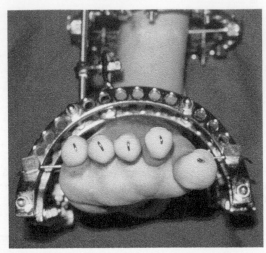

Fig. 10. Postoperative aspect of a right foot after correction of the clawed toe deformities. Note the pins used for temporary transarticular fixation of the toes.

that proper patient compliance with this method of treatment requires thorough patient education on the details of the treatment. Allowing patients to remain in the hospital during the entire course of correction is ideal. This allows for careful supervision and avoids complications to the soft tissue while preserving function of the lower extremity through assisted physical therapy. Although a prolonged hospital stay may raise costs of treatment, it also allows more predictable results and avoids complications that would lead to additional surgery. It also is possible to carefully instruct patients on how to handle the Ilizarov device themselves, but this requires meticulous patient selection and weekly outpatient supervision by a health care team.

The majority of patients who have recurrent clubfoot treated with circular external fixator develop late asymptomatic spontaneous ankylosis of the foot and ankle[18] (**Fig. 13**). Another late sequelae is symptomatic arthritis of the ankle or the midfoot joints, which commonly must be treated with arthrodesis for pain relief.[7] This late

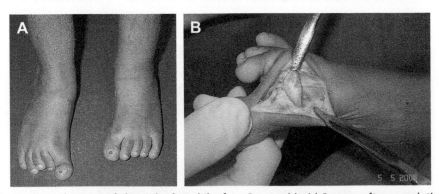

Fig. 11. Frontal aspect of the right foot (*A*) of an 8-year-old girl 3 years after completing correction of a recurrent clubfoot deformity with the modular circular external fixator. Note the varus deformity of the hallux caused by a metatarsal-phalangeal dislocation that was treated with fusion (*B*).

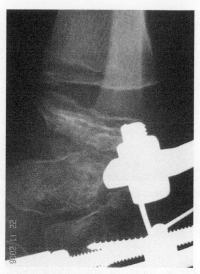

Fig. 12. Lateral radiographic view of the right ankle during correction of recurrent clubfoot with the modular circular external fixator showing dislocation of the distal tibia epiphysis (*arrow*).

arthritis is best interpreted as a result of the realignment of the chronically irregular joint surfaces, which likely are unable to tolerate the stresses of their restored function.

Recurrence of the deformity may take place months or years after complete foot correction. Each component of the deformity can recur separately or in different combinations. The most common are equinocavus, equinovarus, and adduction/supination. The recurrence of the equinus deformity, to a greater or lesser degree, probably is secondary to a lack in bone support to anchor the foot after the Ilizarov device is removed.[6,7,18] Therefore, it is important to use a rigid ankle-foot orthosis until complete stabilization of the foot is achieved after the soft tissue distraction process. Another possible cause for the recurrence of the deformities, especially those in adduction and supination, is the imbalance between the remaining muscular forces, primarily of the anterior and posterior tibial muscles. In such cases, corrective

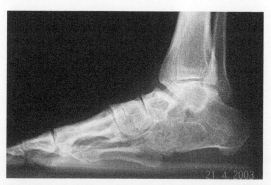

Fig. 13. Lateral standing radiographic view of the right foot, at 84 months' follow-up, showing spontaneous and complete ankylosis of the foot and ankle developed after the treatment of recurrent clubfoot deformity with the modular circular external fixator.

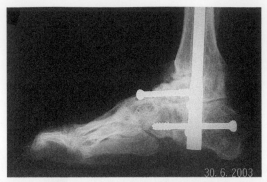

Fig. 14. Lateral standing radiographic view of the right foot, at 36 months' follow-up after the treatment of recurrent clubfoot deformity with the external fixator. Modeling panarthrodesis was performed to treat partial recurrence of the deformities and painful arthritis. The radiograph shows bone fusion of the midfoot and hindfoot in progress.

arthrodesis (midfoot, subtalar, triple, or tibiotalocalcaneal) is indicated for proper alignment and stabilization of moderate or severe residual deformities (**Fig. 14**). Previous correction of the major foot deformities with the external fixator allows technically easier and safer surgeries, avoiding extensive soft tissue dissection and additional shortening of the foot, because only minor bone resection is required during the arthrodesis procedure.

In the authors' opinion, complimentary arthrodesis should not be considered a treatment failure after major correction of recurrent clubfoot deformities with circular external fixator, because these feet already are severely deformed and stiff before the treatment. The final objective of treating a recurred clubfoot is to reach a nonpainful plantigrade foot. This can be achieved successfully in 77% of cases, according to authors' experience.[18] Patients' personal satisfaction is high. Unsatisfactory results are treated with leg or foot orthosis or submitted to traditional corrective surgery (arthrodesis) under more favorable conditions, with fewer risks to patients and to surgeons.

REFERENCES

1. McKay DW. New concept of an approach to clubfoot treatment—evaluation and results. J Pediatr Orthop 1983;3:141–8.
2. Turco VJ. Surgical correction of resistant clubfoot. One-stage posteromedial release with internal fixation. J Bone Joint Surg Am 1971;53-A:477–97.
3. Paley D. The correction of complex foot deformities using Ilizarov's distraction osteotomies. Clin Orthop 1993;293:97–111.
4. Silver L, Grant AD, Atar D, et al. Use of tissue expansion in clubfoot surgery. Foot Ankle 1993;14:117–22.
5. Bradish CF, Noor S. The Ilizarov method in the management of relapsed club feet. J Bone Joint Surg Br 2000;82-B:387–91.
6. Ferreira RC, Stefani KC, Fonseca Filho FF, et al. Correção do pé torto congênito inveterado e recidivado pelo método de Ilizarov. Rev Bras Ortop 1999;34:505–12 [in Portuguese].
7. Ferreira RC, Costa MT, Frizzo GG, et al. Correction of neglected clubfoot using the Ilizarov external fixator. Foot Ankle Int 2006;27:266–73.

8. Grant AD, Atar D, Lehman WB. The Ilizarov technique in correction of complex foot deformities: a preliminary report. Foot Ankle 1990;11:01–5.
9. Grant AD, Atar D, Lehman WB. The Ilizarov technique in correction of complex foot deformities. Clin Orthop 1992;280:94–103.
10. Grill F, Franke J. The Ilizarov distractor for the correction of relapsed or neglected clubfoot. J Bone Joint Surg Br 1987;69-B:593–7.
11. Hosny GA. Correction of foot deformities by the Ilizarov method without corrective osteotomies or soft tissue release. J Pediatr Orthop 2002;11(B):121–8.
12. Huerta de la F. Correction of the neglected clubfoot by the Ilizarov method. Clin Orthop 1994;301:89–93.
13. Ilizarov GA, Shevtsov VI, Kuźmin NV. Method of treating talipes equinocavus. Ortop Travmatol Protez 1983;5:46–8.
14. Koczewski O, Shadi M, Napiontek M. Foot lengthening using the Ilizarov device: the transverse tarsal joint resection versus osteotomy. J Pediatr Orthop 2002; 11(B):68–72.
15. Oganesyan OV, Istomina IS. Talipes equinocavovarus deformities corrected with the aid of a hinged-distraction apparatus. Clin Orthop 1991;266:43–51.
16. Oganesyan OV, Istomina IS, Kuzmin VI. Treatment of equinocavovarus deformity in adults with the use of a hinged distraction apparatus. J Bone Joint Surg Am 1996;78-A:546–56.
17. Wallander H, Hansson G, Tjernströn B. Correction of persistent clubfoot deformities with the Ilizarov external fixator. Acta Orthop Scand 1996;67:283–7.
18. Ferreira RC, Costa MT, Frizzo GG, et al. Correction of severe recurrent clubfoot using a simplified setting of the Ilizarov device. Foot Ankle Int 2007;28:557–68.
19. Flynn JM, Donohoe M, Willian G. Independent assessment of two classification systems. J Pediatr Orthop 1998;18:323–7.
20. Choi IH, Yang MS, Chung CY, et al. The treatment of recurrent arthrogrypotic club foot in children by the Ilizarov method. J Bone Joint Surg Br 2001;83-B:731–7.
21. Hsu KY, Kuo KN, Hsu RW. Correction of foot deformity by Ilizarov method in a patient with Segawa disease. Clin Orthop 1995;314:199–202.

Neuromuscular Deformity: Treatment with External Fixation

Metin Kucukkaya, MD[a],*, Unal Kuzgun, MD[b]

KEYWORDS

- Distraction osteogenesis • Foot deformity • Llizarov method
- Neuromuscular deformity • External fixation

A multiplanar foot deformity is defined by the presence of more than one deformity affecting the foot. These deformities may develop in any plane, including the frontal, sagittal, or transverse planes. This article focuses on the treatment of multiplanar neuromuscular foot deformities with external fixation, reviewing the indications, preoperative planning, techniques, and complications.

Any spastic or paralytic disorder affecting the neuromuscular structure can lead to muscle imbalance and deformity of the foot and ankle.[1–5] Muscle imbalance prevents normal joint motion and may result in various functional disabilities. Initially, muscle imbalance produces a progressive flexible deformity. With skeletal growth, bony deformities may occur secondary to limitations of the soft tissues and joint contractures. If untreated, callus or skin ulceration, stress fractures of the metatarsals, and associated skeletal system problems may develop. The patient may complain of pain, difficulty with shoewear or orthotics, decreased ambulatory capacity, instability, gait abnormalities, and a poor cosmetic appearance.

In the management of a patient with a neuromuscular foot deformity, the patient's age, skeletal maturity at the time of disease onset, and etiology are important for understanding the nature of the deformity. Multiplanar foot deformities may result from a bony deformity, joint or soft tissue contracture, or combination thereof. If the neuromuscular problem begins before skeletal maturity, bone remodeling is affected, and the deformity is more complex. If the neuromuscular problem develops after skeletal maturity, muscle imbalance may cause only joint contracture or subluxation.

The cause of a neuromuscular foot deformity may be either static or progressive in nature.[3,4,6–8] Static causes include cerebral palsy; poliomyelitis; stroke; spinal cord or peripheral nerve injury; traumatic muscle injury; compartment syndrome; or iatrogenic

---

[a] Orthopaedic and Traumatology Department, Sisli Etfal Research and Training Hospital, Guzelbahce sk, Tugrul ap, kat:2, no:33-35, Nisantası, Istanbul, Turkey
[b] Orthopaedic and Traumatology Department, Sisli Etfal Research and Training Hospital, Nilufer sk, Nilufer ap kat:2, Osmanbey, Istanbul, Turkey
* Corresponding author.
E-mail address: mkucukkaya@yahoo.com (M. Kucukkaya).

Foot Ankle Clin N Am 14 (2009) 447–470
doi:10.1016/j.fcl.2009.04.005
1083-7515/09/$ – see front matter © 2009 Elsevier Inc. All rights reserved.

foot.theclinics.com

reasons (injection injury of the sciatic nerve or excessive tendon release during surgical correction for clubfoot). Progressive causes include Charcot-Marie-Tooth disease, muscular dystrophy, syringomyelia, tethered cord, myelomeningocele, and diastema-tomyelia. The progressive nature of these disorders may affect the end results.

Neuromuscular foot deformities are usually accompanied by other problems. Coexisting complicating factors include instability caused by muscle imbalance; sensory impairment; poor soft tissue and bone condition (previous surgery); insufficient ambulatory capability; pre-existing arthrosis; vascular insufficiency; knee and hip contractures; and leg-length discrepancy.

Surgical management is necessary for patients who have a progressive deformity or who have a deformity that causes functional disability. In the treatment of neuromuscular foot deformities, the goal is to provide a painless, plantigrade, stable foot that can fit into a shoe without undue difficulty. In general, the correction of neuromuscular foot deformities has been managed through soft tissue releases, tendon transfers, osteotomies, or arthrodesis.[3,4,6–18] Joint motion should be preserved to the greatest extent possible, particularly in patients with impaired sensation. Before foot maturity, generally at ages younger than 12 years, extra-articular osteotomies and balancing muscle force may be useful to lessen any residual deformity at the time of triple arthrodesis. To prevent the progression of bony deformity in planovalgus feet with a neuromuscular cause, extra-articular subtalar arthrodesis and arthroresis with implants (ie, a staple or peg) are traditionally performed.[19–22] These techniques are applicable, however, in only mild, flexible planovalgus deformities.

In previously operated or severe rigid neuromuscular foot deformities, the tendons, joint capsules, ankle ligaments, and scar tissue within the fat and fascial layers are contracted. In most of these patients, an appropriate correction cannot be obtained with soft tissue procedures alone and osteotomies or fusions are usually required.[23] Previously described methods for arthrodesis and wedge-shaped midfoot osteotomies can be used to treat most of these deformities.[13,24–26] These methods, however, may also reduce the height of the foot, lower the malleoli, and may cause persistent postoperative swelling. They may also create difficulty in fitting shoes. The most commonly reported complications of these procedures are nonunion; residual deformity; recurrent deformity; ankle arthritis; and avascular necrosis of the talus, which may require further surgery.[14,16,27,28] In addition, in cavovarus foot deformities, complete realignment with a Dwyer closing wedge osteotomy can be achieved only in mild hindfoot varus.[29] Although these conventional techniques achieve acute correction of the deformity, they may result in neurovascular injury and soft tissue healing problems.

Although knowledge of pathologic foot anatomy and management methods has increased since the time of Hippocrates, gradual distraction techniques are still important in the first-line treatment of foot deformities, independently of severity.[30–33] In classical hand manipulation techniques, the correcting force is transmitted to the bone over soft tissues. Soft tissues can tolerate only a limited manipulative force. The correction of foot deformities with gradual distraction using an external fixator, however, has been described as an alternative technique.[34–48] Kucukkaya and colleagues[42] reported a series of nine neuromuscular foot deformities treated with the Ilizarov method. In all cases, a combination of midfoot and calcaneal osteotomies was used to obtain a stiff subtalar joint. No major complication was observed, and a painless, stable, plantigrade foot was obtained in all but one patient.

In distraction techniques, the manipulative force is transmitted to the bone directly by Kirschner (K) wires. In this manner, soft tissue complications can be prevented and most rigid foot deformities can be corrected.

Moreover, during correction of the deformity, hand manipulation techniques generate a compression effect in the foot joints, whereas gradual correction with external fixator techniques produces a distraction effect in the foot joints. With the gradual distraction technique, the incisions are usually smaller and extensive periosteal stripping or soft tissue dissection is not required. In the distraction technique, an osteotomy is used instead of bone resection, the height of the foot is not reduced, and shoe-fitting problems are prevented. Although the final correction is achieved intraoperatively with conventional surgical methods, all components of the deformity can be corrected both gradually and independently with the distraction technique. The gradual distraction technique using an external fixator is also amenable to adjustment throughout the treatment period and the amount of correction is always controlled by the surgeon. The gradual osteotomy distraction technique reduces the risk of tissue damage from surgery and provides a stable foot, similar to a triple arthrodesis.

In the gradual distraction technique, the release of contracted soft tissues, such as scars, ligaments, or tendons, is usually not necessary for correction of the deformity. Instead, a continuous distraction force is sufficient to correct most of these deformities. Ligaments and tendons usually become pliant by the time that the external fixator is removed, which may be the result of continuous distraction force during treatment.

GRADUAL DISTRACTION TECHNIQUE

With the gradual distraction technique, there are two ways to correct deformities in the foot: soft tissue distraction and osteotomy distraction.[45,47] With the soft tissue distraction technique, the deformity is corrected through the subluxated joints and physes of immature bones. This technique is preferred in cases with soft tissue and joint contractures, rather than bone deformities, or deformities that are established after foot maturity. In the osteotomy distraction technique, the deformity is corrected through the osteotomy lines. Osteotomy distraction is preferred in cases with bone deformity that occurred before maturity or in patients who have a deformity with arthrosis. In addition, osteotomy distraction is preferred in patients with neuromuscular imbalance. Four basic osteotomy techniques or combinations thereof can be used to correct foot deformities: (1) midfoot, (2) calcaneal, (3) U-shaped, and (4) supramalleolar osteotomies (**Fig. 1**).

The midfoot osteotomy starts from the cuneiform bones, navicular, or neck of the talus at the apex of the deformity and extends to the plantar surface. This procedure is used to correct forefoot deformities. If there is no subtalar joint motion or the goal is a stiff subtalar joint, the osteotomy line crosses the subtalar joint. If subtalar joint motion must be protected, the osteotomy is performed more distally at the cuboid or navicular level. The calcaneal osteotomy is performed between the dorsum of the calcaneal tuberosity and the plantar surface of the foot, and is used to correct hindfoot deformities. The U-shaped osteotomy starts from the neck of the talus, crosses the subtalar joint, and extends to the superior aspect of the tuberosity of the calcaneus. This osteotomy is used in cases in which the apex of the deformity is in the talus or in cases with a normal relationship between the hindfoot and forefoot. U-shaped osteotomy blocks subtalar joint motion and may be used to increase the height of the foot. Finally, a supramalleolar osteotomy is performed in the distal tibial metaphyses, and is preferred in cases exhibiting distal tibial deformity and ankylosed subtalar and tibiotalar joints to obtain a plantigrade foot. In addition, this osteotomy can lengthen the lower extremity.

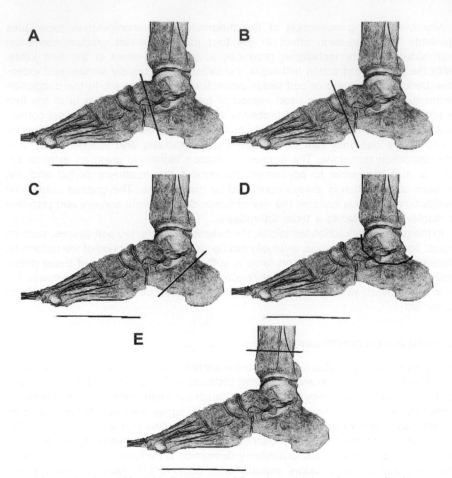

Fig.1. Schematic. The midfoot (*A, B*), calcaneal (*C*), U-shaped (*D*), and supramalleolar osteotomy (*E*). Note the midfoot (*A*) and U-shaped osteotomies (*D*) cross the subtalar joint and produce a stiff foot (see additional explanation in the text).

Combined midfoot and calcaneal osteotomies are usually referred to as a "V-shaped osteotomy"; this procedure allows correction of the anterior and posterior segments in relation to the middle segment. The U-shaped and midfoot osteotomies produce a stiff subtalar joint. The distinct characteristics of these osteotomies are especially important for obtaining a stiff, stable foot in severe neuromuscular foot deformities.

PATIENT EVALUATION AND PREOPERATIVE PLANNING

Preoperative evaluation should include the patient's clinical and family histories, a physical examination, electromyographic and nerve conduction studies, and a radiographic examination of the lower extremities. The patient's age and skeletal maturity at the time of disease onset, progressiveness of the neuromuscular disorder, and compensatory deformities should be evaluated in the preoperative period.

The physical examination should include neurologic and vascular evaluation: gait analysis: inspection of the typical features of the deformity (mid-foot cavus, hind-foot varus, calcaneocavus, and so forth); range of motion measurements; and obtaining a standing footprint. The primary deforming force, muscle strength grade, and any spasticity should be evaluated for possible tendon transfer procedures. Additional complicating factors, such as knee and hip contractures, leg-length discrepancy, sensation problems, and poor soft tissue conditions (previous surgery or bunions), should be considered in the treatment plan. The patient's ambulatory capability should be evaluated preoperatively using a collaborative approach that includes a neurologist, physical therapist, and pediatrician, if necessary.

Compensatory deformities in the foot and ankle are common, because many of the lower extremity deformities can be compensated by the ankle, hindfoot, and forefoot. Frontal and sagittal plane deformities of the distal tibia can usually be compensated by the subtalar and ankle joint, respectively (**Fig. 2**). Similarly, a multiplanar ankle or hindfoot deformity can be compensated by the forefoot. For instance, a hindfoot eversion deformity can be compensated by dorsiflexion of the first metatarsal ray and forefoot supination (**Fig. 3**A). A hindfoot inversion deformity can be compensated by forefoot pronation (see **Fig. 3**B). The flexibility of the hindfoot as it relates to the forefoot is critical in the evaluation. The Coleman block test evaluates the flexibility of the hindfoot and helps to determine the type of surgery.[49]

Radiographs, including weight-bearing anteroposterior, lateral, and posterior tangential radiographs of the foot and ankle are obtained at the initial assessment. Standard radiographs and clinical views are usually sufficient for defining the deformity. Any angulation, rotation, or translation in the coronal, sagittal, or axial planes of both the hindfoot and forefoot should be noted. The talus-first metatarsal angle (Meary's angle), calcaneal-first metatarsal angle (Hibb's angle), and calcaneal pitch angle, which is defined as the angle formed by the intersection of a line drawn tangentially to the inferior surface of the calcaneus and one drawn along the plantar surface of the foot, are measured on lateral weight-bearing radiographs. The posterior tangential radiograph of the foot reveals the position and shape of the calcaneus. If there is a transverse plane rotational deformity of the hindfoot, the calcaneus appears short and deformed in standard lateral radiographs. In this situation, true lateral hindfoot radiographs should be obtained (**Fig. 4**).

Three-dimensional CT is helpful for evaluating degenerative joints and transverse plane rotation–translation deformities of the hindfoot. Three-dimensional CT is also useful to determine the nature of the deformity (bone, soft tissue contracture, or a combination).

Vascular investigations of the patient should also be performed in the preoperative period. Tracing or marking the paths of major arteries on the skin using Doppler ultrasonography is very important in patients with multiplanar foot deformities, or in those who have had previous surgeries that may have displaced or injured neurovascular structures (**Fig. 5**).

TREATMENT STRATEGIES

Development of a treatment strategy is dependent on the individual nature of the deformity and patient characteristics, including age at disease onset (ie, before or after maturity); remaining remodeling capacity; presence of established bone deformity; arthritic changes; and progressiveness of the primary disorders.

Although additional soft tissue releases are usually not necessary for correcting the deformity, a primary plantar fascia release may be performed to prevent intense pain during correction. This is discussed later. If necessary, a tendon transfer may be performed after a fixed deformity correction.

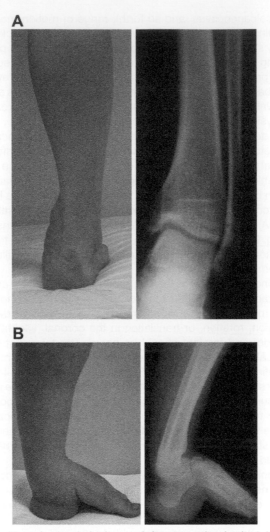

Fig. 2. (*A*) Compensation of a distal tibial varus deformity with subtalar joint valgus. The foot may be plantigrade despite a distal tibial deformity. (*B*) Compensation of the distal tibial sagittal plane deformity with calcaneus and forefoot adaptation.

Another important factor is the nature of the deformity. Multiplanar foot deformities involve some compensatory changes that can be flexible or rigid. An important rule is that if a flexible foot deformity compensates for another rigid foot deformity, the flexible deformity should not be corrected.

Reduced Remaining Remodeling Capacity (Older Patients)

If the patient experienced early disease onset (ie, before maturity), has an established bone deformity, or possesses reduced remodeling capacity (ie, usually in patients older than 8–10 years), osteotomy distraction techniques may be useful as salvage procedures. If there are no arthritic changes, no progressive disease, and the

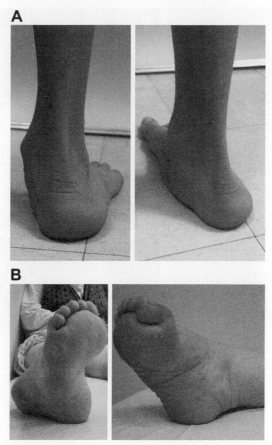

Fig. 3. (*A*) Compensation of a hindfoot eversion deformity with dorsiflexion of the first metatarsal ray and forefoot supination. (*B*) Compensation of a hindfoot inversion deformity with forefoot pronation.

deforming force can be balanced by soft tissue procedures (eg, tendon transfer), the soft tissue distraction technique is preferred in those patients.

If the patient experienced late disease onset (ie, after maturity), joint contracture rather than bone deformity, possesses reduced remodeling capacity, and does not show arthritic changes, soft tissue distraction and elimination of the deforming force (eg, tendon transfer) is preferred. If the patient has progressive disease or the deforming force cannot be balanced, the osteotomy distraction technique is preferred.

Greater Remaining Remodeling Capacity (Younger Patients)

If the patient experienced early disease onset (ie, before maturity) and retains a greater degree of remodeling capacity (ie, usually younger than 8–10 years), soft tissue distraction and a technique that balances the deforming force should be used. If the patient has a progressive disease or the deforming force cannot be balanced, osteotomy distraction techniques are preferred.

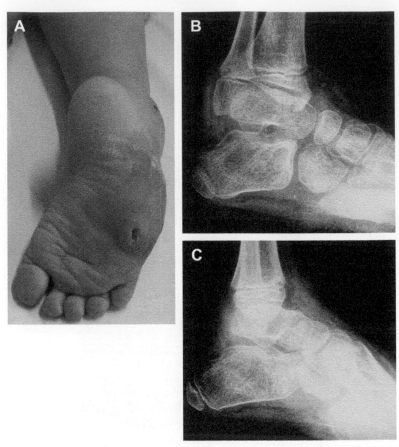

Fig. 4. (*A*) Plantar view of an equinovarus deformity in a patient with myelomeningocel. Note the transverse plane rotational deformity of the hindfoot. (*B*) The calcaneus appears short and deformed in standard lateral radiograph. (*C*) True lateral hindfoot radiograph reveals correct calcaneal length.

PREPARING THE EXTERNAL FIXATOR

An external fixator that mimics the foot deformity is usually constructed intraoperatively. Two types of frames can be designed: a hinged or constrained frame; or an unhinged, unconstrained frame. In the hinged frame design, the deformity is corrected around the hinge axis. In the correction of neuromuscular foot deformities, hinges are usually necessary to prevent uncontrolled correction, which can occur because of muscle imbalance. In contrast, the joints of the foot and ankle serve as the hinge in an unconstrained design. An unconstrained frame is useful for soft tissue distraction, such as the correction of a pure equinus deformity.

The external fixator consists of three main parts: (1) a base, which is placed on the leg; (2) a heel; and (3) forefoot parts. The base is composed of a ring and a square frame that fix the tibia. Both the ring and square frame have one K-wire and one Schanz pin. The distal frame of the base part should be a square frame to allow face-to-face connection of holes with the square frame of the heel part. This design allows perfect placement of the hinges. If there are additional deformities requiring correction, such as a leg-length discrepancy or joint contractures, a base is

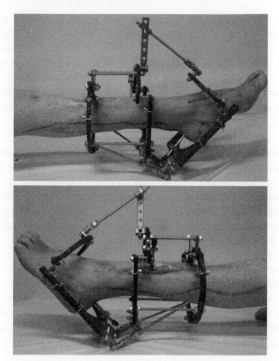

Fig. 5. Marking the major arteries on the skin preoperatively using Doppler ultrasonography.

constructed for these deformities. The heel and forefoot parts are made of radiolucent material to obtain the best postoperative radiologic images. In addition, parts of the forefoot frame can be removed during correction, if necessary. Two crossed olive wires or a single K-wire combined with a single Schanz pin is used on the heel part. The forefoot part of the frame usually consists of two parallel half rings. In severely deformed feet, two full rings can be used to obtain a more stable construct. One K-wire is inserted through the first and fifth metatarsals distally, and one K-wire is placed as close as possible to the midfoot osteotomy. With a U-shaped osteotomy or a combination of midfoot and calcaneal osteotomies, a triangular middle bone segment is created within the bodies of the talus and calcaneus. This mobile bone segment should be stabilized with one K-wire or a Schanz pin, and connected to the lower ring of the base frame, to enable correction of the anterior and posterior segments relative to the middle segment.

The correction of transverse plane rotational deformities of the hindfoot using an Ilizarov external fixator is difficult. Perfect placement of the complex hinge system needed for rotational correction relative to the holes on the square foot frame is usually problematic.[50] Computer-assisted external fixator systems, such as the Taylor Spatial Frame (Smith & Nephew Richards, Memphis, TN, USA), are very useful, but complicated devices for the correction of these deformities.[44,48] The correction of rotational deformities of the hindfoot using a Taylor Spatial Frame or in combination with a classical circular external fixator system is very effective.

SURGICAL METHOD

Surgery should be performed under general or epidural anesthesia without neuromuscular blockade. A radiolucent operating table and image intensifier are necessary.

After applying the base part of the frame, the tourniquet is inflated and osteotomy is performed. If necessary, the tarsal tunnel should be decompressed before completing the osteotomy. A lateral incision and osteotome are used for the U-shaped and calcaneal osteotomies. The sural nerve must be identified and protected while performing these osteotomies. The drill osteotome technique is used for a supramalleolar osteotomy. The Gigli saw technique is used for a midfoot osteotomy (**Fig. 6**). A Gigli saw osteotomy can be performed before applying the base part of the frame and involves three or four small incisions.[42,46] A 0.5-cm incision is made through the lateral aspect of the talar neck, under image intensifier control. From this incision, a long curved hemostat is passed between the dorsal aspect of the talar neck and extensor tendons. Another 0.5-cm incision is made between the lateral border of the tibialis posterior tendon and the medial aspect of the talar neck. This second incision should be made over the end of the curved hemostat that was passed through the first incision. The Gigli saw is grasped and pulled away from the second incision using this hemostat. One or two additional incisions are necessary at the plantar aspect of these incisions. The distal end of the calcaneal osteotomy incision can be used as the fourth incision. The Gigli saw is used around the talar neck and anterior part of the calcaneus in a similar manner. After checking the position of the Gigli saw with an image intensifier, the osteotomy is completed. The midfoot and calcaneal osteotomies are compressed and fixed with a temporary K-wire to prevent bleeding. After closing the incisions, the tourniquet is deflated. The remaining forefoot and heel parts of an external fixator that mimics the deformity are applied. The frame is connected using universal hinges and rods depending on whether they are to function as a distractor or compressor.

AFTERCARE

Correction begins on the second postoperative day, and should proceed as rapidly as soft tissue adaptation and patient tolerance allows. The goal of the distraction

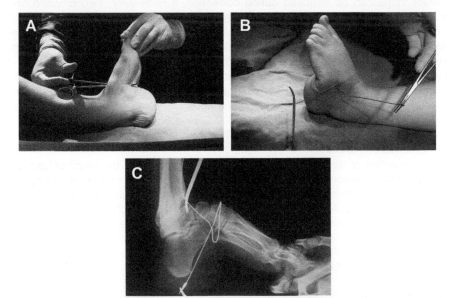

Fig. 6. The Gigli saw technique. (*A, B*) The Gigli saw is grasped and pulled away from the small incisions using a hemostat. (*C*) The position of the Gigli saw is checked with an image intensifier or radiograph (see additional explanation in the text).

procedure is to obtain a 1 to 1.5 mm/day opening at the osteotomy site. Physical therapy begins 2 days postoperatively with gait, lower extremity motion, and phalanx-stretching exercises. Pin site care is performed twice a week with hydrogen peroxide and saline for the foot and fixator. If early signs of pin site infection are observed, such as localized redness, pain, tenderness, warmth, swelling, and drainage, then distraction is stopped and pin care is increased to twice daily. If these symptoms do not improve rapidly, oral antibiotics are started for a minimum of 7 days. The external fixator is kept in the locked position for 6 additional weeks after the correction period, which usually requires 2 to 4 weeks according to the nature of the deformity. The frame is then removed and a cast applied under general anesthesia. Full weight-bearing is permitted as soon as possible with a cast.

The foot is usually completely pliant at the time of frame removal, likely secondary to the effect of the continuous distraction force on the soft tissues. This may allow for the correction of any residual deformity; even a limited overcorrection may be performed. The cast should be replaced in 1 to 2 weeks with one that fits after the swelling has

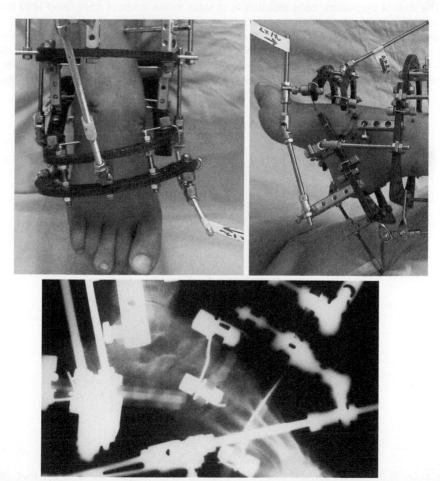

Fig. 7. Placement of the K-wire as closely as possible to the osteotomy sites to prevent premature consolidation.

resolved and the cast becomes loose. To prevent recurrence of the deformity, the patient should be protected with a cast and orthotics for a sufficient period to allow complete adaptation of the soft tissues. The first 6 to 8 weeks of the protection should be done with cast, the rest of time can be continued with orthotics. If the deformity was established before skeletal maturity, the foot should be protected for a minimum of 1 year. If it occurred after maturity, a minimum of 6 months of protection is sufficient. If the underlying neuromuscular disease is progressive, the protection time should be increased.

PROBLEMS AND COMPLICATIONS

In the foot, the risks of premature consolidation, soft tissue problems, intense pain, neurovascular injury, and recurrence of the deformity are greater than for other parts of the body.[42,44] In addition, toe contractures, pin tract problems, physeal disruption, and psychologic intolerance are common during the treatment of foot deformities with an external fixator.[34,36–41,46,51]

The risk of premature consolidation is greater in the midfoot compared with the other bones, whereas this problem is rarely observed in the hindfoot. There are four causes of premature consolidation. The first is an incomplete osteotomy, which can be prevented with the Gigli saw technique. The second is incorrect placement of the forefoot K-wire. If the forefoot K-wire is away from the midfoot osteotomy site, a distraction gap may be created in the joint space instead of the osteotomy site.

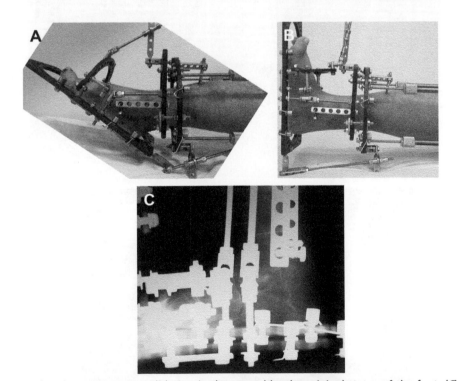

Fig. 8. (*A, B*) Premature consolidation is also caused by the original status of the foot. (*C*) Decreased consolidation is apparent. The distraction rate must be balanced between soft tissues and bone (see additional explanation in the text).

The K-wire must be placed as closely as possible to the osteotomy site to prevent this complication (**Fig. 7**). The third reason for premature consolidation is insufficient stabilization of the mobile triangular middle bone segment that is created within the bodies of the talus and calcaneus. Occasionally, one K-wire is insufficient and the K-wire connection may cause trouble. In this case, stabilization of the segment using a Schanz pin is helpful. Finally, premature consolidation may also be caused by the original status of the foot. If the distraction rate is regulated for the osteotomy site, excessive soft tissue distraction may result in soft tissue necrosis. If the distraction rate is regulated for the soft tissues, the osteotomy site may consolidate prematurely (**Fig. 8**). Consequently, the distraction rate must be balanced between the appropriate rates for soft tissues and bone, according to the patient's tolerance. The authors begin correction on the second postoperative day instead of the fifth day, and proceed as rapidly as possible while considering both soft tissue adaptation and the patient's tolerance.

Toe contractures are another common problem when treating foot deformities with an external fixator. Toe contracture and metatarsophalangeal subluxation may develop in any plane, according to nature of the deformity, including dorsal, plantar, and medial contractures.[43] Although plantar toe contractures occur primarily during the correction of equinus and cavus deformities, dorsal toe contractures occur during the correction of dorsiflexion deformities. In severe neuromuscular foot deformities, physical therapy is usually ineffective because of the muscle imbalance. To prevent this problem, slings, orthosis, or temporary K-wire fixation may be used; otherwise, tendon lengthening or tenotomies are inevitable.

The authors' approach to toe contractures in children is different from that in adults. Joint luxation does not occur in the metatarsophalangeal joints of children, even in serious contractures during deformity correction. Children may not cooperate fully with physical therapy programs. During frame removal and cast application under general anesthesia, the phalanx can easily be corrected acutely with hand

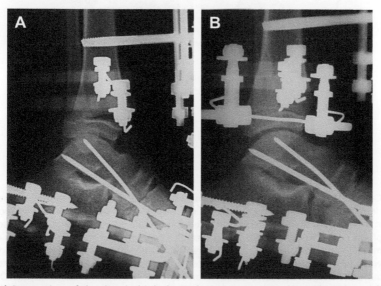

Fig. 9. (*A*) Separation of the distal tibial physis during correction. (*B*) Reducing and fixing of this separation using a K-wire.

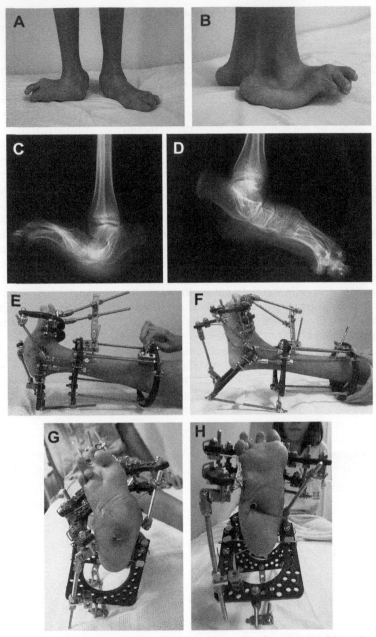

Fig. 10. Case 1. (*A–D*) Preoperative views and radiographs of a 10-year-old myelomeningocele patient with a bilateral rocker-bottom deformity. (*E–H*) During gradual correction of the right foot deformity, the K-wire that fixed the mobile triangular middle bone segment from a plantar site through the tibia to correct the anterior and posterior segments relative to the middle segment sunk into the plantar skin. Note that a completely hinged frame design was used. The deformity was corrected from the midfoot and calcaneal osteotomy lines around the hinge axis. (*I, J*) Gradually correction of the left foot deformity. (*K–O*) Views and radiographs after protection with orthotics for 1 year.

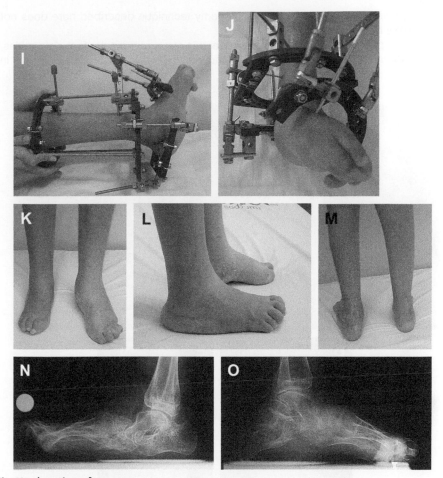

Fig. 10. (*continued*)

manipulation in children. Routine protection with a cast and orthotics (4–6 weeks minimum) is enough to prevent the recurrence of phalanx contracture.

Recurrence of the deformity is a common problem when using distraction treatment for foot deformities,[38,51] and the risk of recurrence increases in cases with congenital problems, progressive disorders, burn contractures, or neuromuscular imbalance.[44] After correcting the neuromuscular foot deformity with distraction treatment, long-term protection with orthotics and muscle balance are required to prevent recurrence. Short-term protection is successful only in cases with acquired deformity after maturity.

The development of avascular necrosis of the talus in the surgical management of foot deformities is controversial. Huber and colleagues[52] evaluated idiopathic clubfoot patients who had undergone a talar neck osteotomy to correct the residual forefoot deformity. These cases were treated with open surgery and a closing wedge osteotomy of the lateral aspect of the talar neck. They suggested that the talar neck osteotomy is responsible for the development of avascular necrosis of the talus, especially in patients under 10 years of age, and proposed that this technique should be abandoned. The authors have yet to observe this complication after distraction treatment, however, perhaps because the Gigli osteotomy technique described here does not compromise blood supply to the talus.

Excessive pain may occur during the correction of neuromuscular foot deformities, even if external fixator principles are followed exactly. Intense pain usually occurs in

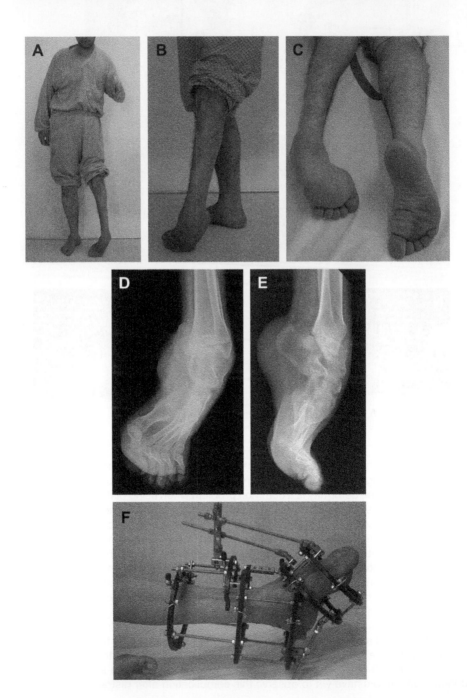

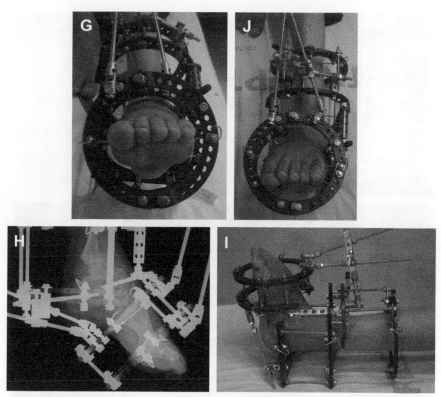

Fig. 11. (*continued*)

cases involving longitudinal arch lengthening, such as in pes cavus deformities. In such cases, the plantar fascia should be released prophylactically at the time of fixator application.

Neurovascular injuries may be caused during pin insertion, during osteotomy, or with rapid distraction. A solid understanding of safe anatomic planes is needed to prevent this complication. Neurovascular structures may be displaced or injured, however, in a previously operated foot or in congenital deformities. In these cases,

◀—————————————————————————————————————

Fig. 11. Case 2. (*A–E*) Preoperative views and radiographs of an equinovarus deformity in a 36-year-old spastic hemiplegic patient. (*F, G*) Acute correction of the hindfoot deformity with a percutaneous Achilles' tenotomy and gradual correction of the forefoot deformity were performed. The forefoot frame was connected to the base and heel frames with two plantar and two anterior rods. The forefoot deformity was corrected around the anterolateral universal hinge axis. This allowed locking of the other rod and hinge connections. (*H*) Postoperative lateral radiograph shows the midfoot osteotomy line and corrected hindfoot deformity. Note that the talus was fixed with a Schanz pin and connected to the lower ring of the base frame. (*I, J*) The anterior part of the proximal forefoot ring was cut and removed to prevent impingement of the Schanz pin that fixed the talus during correction. Cutting the forefoot frame did not result in fixator failure because a full ring was used instead of a half-ring. (*K*) Lateral radiograph after correction. (*L–P*) Views and radiographs after protection for 10 months with a cast and orthotics.

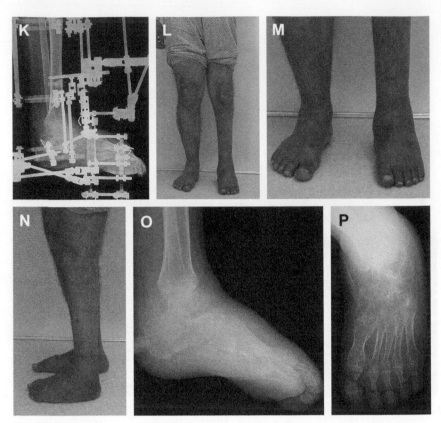

Fig. 11. (*continued*)

the major arteries should be marked on the skin preoperatively using Doppler ultrasonography (see **Fig. 5**). This step reduces the risk of iatrogenic injury to a neurovascular structure. In addition, posterior tibial nerve injury may follow either acute or gradual correction or during an osteotomy.[42,44–46] In the gradual distraction technique, the risk of posterior tibial nerve injury at the tarsal tunnel is anticipated in cases involving the correction of hindfoot varus, ankle equinus, and previous scar tissue.[53] The authors no longer perform routine tarsal tunnel decompression unless the posterior tibial nerve is at risk.

Distal tibial physeal separation may occur during the correction of foot deformities in children. This rare complication is primarily observed during equinus correction when an unhinged frame is used. In children, the distal physis is vulnerable and may not tolerate excessive force during correction. When this problem occurs, the distal epiphysis should be reduced and fixed with a K-wire (**Fig. 9**).

CASE PRESENTATION AND DISCUSSION
Case Example 1

A 10-year-old patient presented with a bilateral rigid rocker-bottom deformity of the foot related to a myelomeningocele (**Fig. 10**). The patient had no obvious ulceration, because she was unable to walk without crutches. Coexisting complicating factors included a sensory deficit, loss of proprioception, bilateral hip dislocations, and metabolic imbalance resulting from renal impairment. A collaborative preoperative assessment found the patient's ambulatory capacity to be sufficient.

Myelomeningoceles may cause many types of foot deformity that are not correlated with the level of spinal involvement.[3,6,54,55] The most frequent deformities are equinus and calcaneus, followed by valgus, clubfoot, and vertical talus. A rocker-bottom deformity in a myelomeningocele that limits the weight-bearing contact surface of the sole may cause ulceration. Serial cast treatment has been recommended, but passive correction of the deformity is impossible. These patients usually require surgical treatment. Surgery is typically delayed until the patient's neurodevelopment allows orthotic ambulation. Triple arthrodesis is an excellent alternative salvage surgical technique for severe deformities at this age.[3] In these cases, the rigid planovalgus position of the foot, the prominence of the talar head medially, and the sensory deficit make the use of orthotics very difficult.

In this particular case, the risk of recurrence was high because she had a severe bone deformity, low remodeling capacity, and no possibility of tendon transfer procedures. In addition, the sensory deficit and metabolic imbalance increased the risk of wound healing problems. Distraction treatment with midfoot and calcaneal osteotomies was chosen. The deformity was corrected gradually around the axis of the hinges from the osteotomy sites. A midfoot osteotomy that crossed to the subtalar joint produced a stiff foot, like a triple arthrodesis, and prevented recurrence.

In this case, the mobile triangular middle bone segment between the midfoot and calcaneus osteotomies was fixed using a free K-wire from a plantar site through the tibia to correct the anterior and posterior segments relative to the middle segment. During deformity correction, this K-wire sank into the plantar skin. Both feet were treated similarly and protected with orthotics to support the soft tissues for 1 year to allow complete adaptation and prevent recurrence of the deformity. Orthotics were preferred over casts to facilitate observation and prevent any skin problems that might have resulted from her sensory impairment.

Case Example 2

This 36-year-old patient had rigid equinovarus and left hand deformities caused by cerebral palsy (**Fig. 11**). He was born with normal-looking feet and hands. He had meningitis at 2 years of age, which resulted in spastic hemiplegia. He had been left untreated. Contractures and fixed foot and hand deformities developed as he grew.

Hemiplegia is primarily observed in the spastic type of cerebral palsy. The weakness usually predominates in the distal aspect of the limb. The upper extremity is usually more severely involved than the lower extremity and equinus and varus are the most common foot deformities in spastic hemiplegia. Most conservative and surgical treatment methods aim to prevent the development of deformities in cerebral palsy. Untreated or residual deformities can be managed only by salvage surgical techniques, however, such as a triple arthrodesis, talectomy, or Ilizarov distraction osteotomies.[3,4,6,13,42,56]

In this case, the hindfoot equinus and varus deformities were corrected acutely with a percutaneous Achilles' tenotomy and fixed with the heel part of the external fixator. In addition, the forefoot equinus, supination, and adductus deformities were corrected gradually from the midfoot osteotomy. After frame removal and cast application, full weight-bearing was allowed. The foot was protected with orthotics for an additional year to allow complete adaptation of the soft tissues and prevent recurrence.

Case Example 3

Poliomyelitis is an acute viral infection that predominantly affects the anterior horn cells in the spinal cord. Necrosis of these cells results in a loss of motor innervation of muscles. The initial goals of treatment include preventing deformity and producing muscle balance. The bone and soft tissue deformities are treated with soft tissue

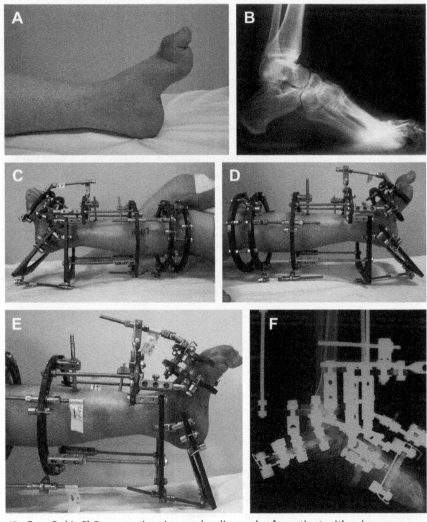

Fig. 12. Case 3. (*A, B*) Preoperative view and radiograph of a patient with calcaneocavus and claw-toes deformities of the foot and a 4-cm leg length discrepancy caused by poliomyelitis. (*C, D*) Calcaneal and midfoot osteotomies were performed for the foot deformity. The percutaneous plantar fascia release incision on the medial-plantar side is visible. This was performed to prevent the intense pain that may occur during the correction of cavus foot. (*E*) Views after correcting the foot deformity and lengthening the tibia by 4 cm. Correction occurred around the axis of the hinges. Stretched plantar skin and toe contracture are seen. (*F*) Radiograph obtained during treatment. (*G–J*) Views and radiographs after treatment. The foot was protected with orthotics for 6 months after frame removal.

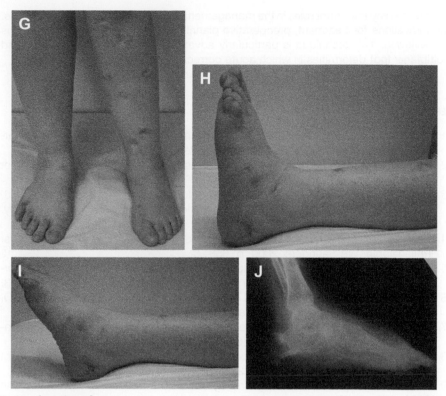

Fig. 12. (*continued*)

releases, tendon transfers, osteotomies, and arthrodeses according to the severity of the deformity and patient age. Deformity correction and joint stability are usually performed with arthrodesis after the age of 10 to 12 years. A calcaneocavus deformity is usually treated with a calcaneal osteotomy combined with the release of the intrinsic muscle and plantar fascia.

A 22-year-old patient had calcaneocavus and claw-toes deformities of the foot. She also had a 4-cm leg-length discrepancy related to poliomyelitis (**Fig. 12**). She had difficulty wearing shoes and limped because of the leg-length discrepancy. In this case, a posterior calcaneal osteotomy and midfoot osteotomy were chosen to correct the foot deformity. A percutaneous plantar fascia release was performed to prevent the intense pain that may occur during the correction of the cavus foot. A tibial osteotomy was added to lengthen the tibia. Hinges were placed at the apex of the osteotomies. The foot deformity was corrected gradually around the axis of the hinges, which produced an opening wedge from the osteotomy sites. In addition, 3 cm of tibial lengthening were obtained at the tibial osteotomy. The foot was protected with orthotics for an additional 6 months to prevent recurrence.

SUMMARY

This article focuses on the treatment of multiplanar neuromuscular foot deformities with external fixation. The treatment of other foot deformities, such as clubfoot or burn contractures, is not discussed. External fixators and gradual distraction techniques play important roles in the management of neuromuscular foot deformities. The indications for treatment, preoperative planning, techniques, and complications are reviewed. This technique is particularly advantageous in neglected or relapsed multiplanar foot deformities in which acute correction may be dangerous.

REFERENCES

1. Alexander IJ, Johnson KA. Assessment and management of pes cavus in Charcot-Marie-Tooth disease. Clin Orthop Relat Res 1989;246:273–81.
2. Beals TC, Nickisch F. Charcot-Marie-Tooth disease and the cavovarus foot. Foot Ankle Clin 2008;13(2):259–74.
3. Dehne R. Congenital and acquired neurologic disorders. In: Coughlin MJ, Their SO, editors. Surgery of the foot and ankle. 8th edition. Philadelphia: Mosby; 2007. p. 1761–806.
4. Dravaric DM. Cerebral palsy. In: Myerson MS, editor. Foot and ankle disorders. Philadelphia: WB Saunders; 2000. p. 658–72.
5. Frawley PA, Broughton NS, Menelaus MB. Incidence and type of hindfoot deformities in patients with low-level spina bifida. J Pediatr Orthop 1998;18(3):312–3.
6. Horstmann HM. Neuromuscular foot deformities in children. In: Gould JS, Their SO, editors. Operative foot surgery. Philadelphia: WB Saunders; 1994. p. 797–833.
7. Mann RA. Charcot-Marie-Tooth disease. In: Gould JS, Their SO, editors. Operative foot surgery. Philadelphia: WB Saunders; 1994. p. 177–83.
8. Marks RM. Midfoot and forefoot issues cavovarus foot: assessment and treatment issues. Foot Ankle Clin 2008;13(2):229–41.
9. Aminian A, Sangeorzan BJ. The anatomy of cavus foot deformity. Foot Ankle Clin 2008;13(2):191–8.
10. Klaue K. Hindfoot issues in the treatment of the cavovarus foot. Foot Ankle Clin 2008;13(2):221–7.
11. Krause FG, Wing KJ, Younger AS. Neuromuscular issues in cavovarus foot. Foot Ankle Clin 2008;13(2):243–58.
12. Lee MC, Sucato DJ. Pediatric issues with cavovarus foot deformities. Foot Ankle Clin 2008;13(2):199–219.
13. Muir D, Angliss RD, Nattrass GR. Tibiocalcaneal arthrodesis for severe calcaneovalgus deformity in cerebral palsy. J Pediatr Orthop 2005;25(5):651–6.
14. Pell RF, Myerson MS, Schon LC. Clinical outcome after primary triple arthrodesis. J Bone Joint Surg Am 2000;82(1):47–57.
15. Rathjen KE, Mubarak SJ. Calcaneal-cuboid-cuneiform osteotomy for the correction of valgus foot deformities in children. J Pediatr Orthop 1998;18(6):775–82.
16. Saltzman CL, Fehrle MJ, Cooper RR, et al. Triple arthrodesis: twenty-five and forty-four year average follow-up of the same patients. J Bone Joint Surg Am 1999;81(10):1391–402.
17. Schwend RM, Drennan JC. Cavus foot deformity in children. J Am Acad Orthop Surg 2003;11(3):201–11.
18. Wines AP, Chen D, Lynch B, et al. Foot deformities in children with hereditary motor and sensory neuropathy. J Pediatr Orthop 2005;25(2):241–4.
19. Crawford AH, Kucharzyk D, Roy DR, et al. Subtalar stabilization of the planovalgus foot by stable arthroereisis in young children who have neuromuscular problems. J Bone Joint Surg Am 1990;72:840–5.
20. Grice DS. An extra-articular arthrodesis of the subastragalar joint for correction of paralytic flat feet in children. J Bone Joint Surg Am 1952;34:927–40.

21. Sanchez AA, Rathjen KE, Mubarak S. Subtalar stable arthroereisis for planoval-gus foot deformity in children with neuromuscular disease. J Pediatr Orthop 1999;19(1):34–8.
22. Vedantam R, Capelli AM, Schoenecker PL. Subtalar arthroereisis for the correc-tion of planovalgus foot in children with neuromuscular disorders. J Pediatr Orthop 1998;18(3):294–8.
23. Levitt RL, Canale ST, Cooke AJ, et al. The role of foot surgery in progressive neuromuscular disorders in children. J Bone Joint Surg Am 1973;55(7):1396–410.
24. Cole WH. Treatment of claw-foot. J Bone Joint Surg 1940;22:895–908.
25. Jahss MH. Evaluation of the cavus foot for operative treatment. Clin Orthop Relat Res 1983;181:52–63.
26. Japas LM. Surgical treatment of pes cavus by tarsal V-osteotomy: preliminary method. J Bone Joint Surg Am 1968;50:927–44.
27. Haddad SL, Myerson MS, Pell RF, et al. Clinical and radiological outcome of revi-sion surgery for failed triple arthrodesis. Foot Ankle Int 1997;18(8):489–99.
28. Wapner KL. Triple arthrodesis in adults. J Am Acad Orthop Surg 1988;5:188–96.
29. Dwyer FC. The present status of the problems of pes cavus. Clin Orthop Relat Res 1975;106:254–75.
30. Herzenberg JE, Radler C, Bor N. Ponseti versus traditional methods of casting for idiopathic clubfoot. J Pediatr Orthop 2002;22(4):517–21.
31. Ponseti IV, Zhivkov M, Davis N. Treatment of the complex idiopathic clubfoot. Clin Orthop Relat Res 2006;451:171–6.
32. Richards BS, Johnston CE, Wilson H. Nonoperative clubfoot treatment using the French physical therapy method. J Pediatr Orthop 2005;25:98–102.
33. Scher DM. The Ponseti method for treatment of congenital club foot. Curr Opin Pediatr 2006;18:22–5.
34. Beaman DN, Gellman R. The basics of ring external fixator application and care. Foot Ankle Clin 2008;13(1):15–27.
35. Bradish CF, Noor S. The Ilizarov method in the management of relapsed clubfeet. J Bone Joint Surg Am 2000;82:387–91.
36. Burns JK, Sullivan R. Correction of severe residual clubfoot deformity in adoles-cent with the Ilizarov technique. Foot Ankle Clin 2004;9(3):571–82.
37. Franke J, Grill F, Hein G, et al. Correction of clubfoot relapse using Ilizarov's appa-ratus in children 8–15 years old. Arch Orthop Trauma Surg 1990;110:33–7.
38. Freedman JA, Watts H, Otsuka NY. The Ilizarov method for the treatment of resis-tant clubfoot: Is it an effective solution. J Pediatr Orthop 2006;26(4):432–7.
39. Grand AD, Atar D, Lehman WB. The Ilizarov technique in correction of complex foot deformities. Clin Orthop Relat Res 1992;280:94–103.
40. Grill F, Franke J. The Ilizarov distractor for the correction of relapsed or neglected clubfoot. J Bone Joint Surg Br 1987;69:593–7.
41. Huerta F. Correction of neglected clubfoot by the Ilizarov method. Clin Orthop Re-lat Res 1994;301:89–93.
42. Kucukkaya M, Kabukcuoglu Y, Kuzgun U. Management of the neuromuscular foot deformities with the Ilizarov method. Foot Ankle Int 2002;23:135–41.
43. Kucukkaya M, Kabukcuoglu Y, Kuzgun U. Correcting and lengthening of meta-tarsal deformity with circular external fixator by distraction osteotomy: a case of longitudinal epiphyseal bracket. Foot Ankle Int 2002;23:427–32.
44. Kucukkaya M. Treatment of complex foot deformities with the Ilizarov distraction method. Türkiye Klinikleri J Surg Med Sci 2007;3(39):101–6.
45. Paley D. The corrections of complex foot deformities using Ilizarov's distraction osteotomies. Clin Orthop Relat Res 1993;293:97–111.

46. Paley D, Herzenberg JE. Application of external fixation to foot and ankle reconstruction. In: Meyerson MS, Their SO, editors. Foot and ankle disorders. Philadelphia: WB Saunders; 2000. p. 1135–88.
47. Paley D, Lamm BM. Correction of the cavus foot using external fixation. Foot Ankle Clin 2004;9(3):611–24.
48. Taylor JC. Perioperative planning for two and three plane deformities. Foot Ankle Clin 2008;13:69–121.
49. Coleman SS, Chesnut WJ. A simple test for hindfoot flexibility in the cavovarus foot. Clin Orthop Relat Res 1977;123:60–2.
50. Kirienko A, Villa A, Calhoun JH. Ilizarov technique for complex foot and ankle deformities. New York-Basel: Marcel Decker; 2004. p. 59–84.
51. Carmichael KD, Maxwell SC, Calhoun JH. Recurrence rates of burn contracture ankle equinus and other foot deformities in children treated with Ilizarov fixation. J Pediatr Orthop 2005;25:523–8.
52. Huber H, Galantay R, Dutoit M. Avascular necrosis after osteotomy of the talar neck to correct residual club-foot deformity in children. J Bone Joint Surg Br 2002;84(3):426–30.
53. Lamm BM, Paley D, Testani M, et al. Tarsal tunnel decompression in leg lengthening and deformity correction of the foot and ankle. J Foot Ankle Surg 2007; 46(3):201–6.
54. Broughton NS, Graham G, Menelaus MB. The high incidence of foot deformity in patients with high-level spina bifida. J Bone Joint Surg Br 1994;76(4):548–50.
55. Frischhut B, Stockl B, Landauer F. Foot deformities in adolescents and young adults with spina bifida. J Pediatr Orthop B 2000;9(3):161–9.
56. Yoo WJ, Chin YC, In HC, et al. Calcaneal lengthening for the planovalgus foot deformity in children with cerebral palsy. J Pediatr Orthop 2005;25(6):781–5.

Cavovarus Foot Reconstruction

Cristian Ortiz, MD[a,b,*], Emilio Wagner, MD[a,b,c], Andres Keller, MD[a,b,c]

KEYWORDS

• Foot • Cavus • Surgery • Treatment • Reconstruction

Cavovarus deformity is defined by fixed equinus of the forefoot on the hind foot, resulting in a pathologic elevation of the longitudinal arch, with either a fixed or flexible varus hind foot deformity. This entity is prevalent in approximately 25% of the population and involves a whole spectrum of deformities that require different approaches to correct them.

The presence of a cavus foot often may be the presenting sign of an underlying neurologic disorder. The most common is a form of hereditary sensory motor neuropathy (HSMN) known as Charcot Marie tooth (CMT) polyneuropathy. A thorough clinical and radiographic examination is mandatory to determine the appropriate final treatment for each patient. Failure to recognize an underlying neurologic disorder may result in use of inappropriate surgical treatment and ultimate recurrence and failure of the reconstruction.

Treatment typically begins with nonsurgical measures; however, in progressive deformities, surgical procedures must be performed soon in a staged protocol to avoid progression of the malalignment and more difficult and less satisfactory solutions. The surgical techniques that must be selected for each patient include soft tissue procedures, osteotomies, and arthrodesis.

This article presents a surgical protocol for surgical reconstruction from the subtle cavus foot described by Manoli[1] to the most complicated cases. The goal is to merge together the available surgical options in a comprehensive way to guide surgical decisions.

ETIOLOGY

The most important reason to investigate the etiology of cavus foot is to determine if the deformity is progressive or static. The most common form of progressive neurologic disorders is CMT,[2,3] which presents in a spectrum of deformities. The probability

---

[a] Foot and Ankle Surgery, Clinica Alemana, Vitacura 5951, Santiago, Chile
[b] Universidad del Desarrollo, Vitacura 5951, Santiago, Chile
[c] Padre Hurtado Hospital, Vitacura 5951, Santiago, Chile
* Corresponding author. Foot and Ankle Surgery, Clinica Alemana, Vitacura 5951, Santiago, Chile.
E-mail address: cortiz@alemana.cl (C. Ortiz).

Foot Ankle Clin N Am 14 (2009) 471–487
doi:10.1016/j.fcl.2009.03.006
1083-7515/09/$ – see front matter © 2009 Elsevier Inc. All rights reserved.

foot.theclinics.com

of a patient who has bilateral cavovarus feet being diagnosed with CMT, regardless of family history, is 78%.[4] Unilateral cavus foot must direct the investigation of the etiology to diseases that cause asymmetrical involvement such as trauma, tumor, or local neurologic damage (**Fig. 1**). Other progressive neurologic disorders include spinal cord lesions such as myelodysplasia, spinal dysraphism, and syringomyelia. Classic static neurologic disorders include cerebral palsy and poliomyelitis.[5]

The most studied type of cavus foot is in patients who have CMT, and for these patients, the deformity manifests in the growing child with the consequent change in shape and position of bones. The muscle involvement progresses from distal to proximal, affecting primarily the tibialis anterior and peroneus brevis, with secondary dysfunction of the intrinsic muscles. Relative sparing of extensor hallucis longus is observed. The relative weakness of the anterior tibialis relative to the peroneus longus results in plantar flexion of the first metatarsal. Secondary to weakness of the tibialis, anterior recruitment of extensor hallucis longus occurs, resulting in cock up deformity of the first toe, with further depression of the metatarsal head and plantar contracture. The forefoot cavus deformity forces the hind foot into varus. The deformity of the hind foot initially is flexible, but can become rigid over time.

Decreased strength of the intrinsic muscles results in unopposed action of the extrinsic musculature (extensor digitorum longus and flexor digitorum longus). This increases equinus and results in claw toes.[5,6] The differential is described in **Box 1**.[7–9]

CLINICAL EXAMINATION

Patients should be examined seated facing the examiner; the examination also should include standing and observed walking. A common and evident finding on physical examination is the peek-a-boo sign described by Manoli.[1] This sign is present when one can see the medial aspect of the heel from the front, as can be seen in **Fig. 2**. This sign is not present when there is valgus or neutral hindfoot position. Some other findings are: hindfoot varus, claw toes, and an elevated arch. The presence of calf atrophy should be observed, and drop foot and balance while walking. Achilles contracture must be evaluated with the Silfverskiöld test. If contracture (inability to dorsiflex past 90°) is observed only with extension of the knee, a gastrocnemius contracture is diagnosed, and it should be treated by a proximal gastrocnemius recession. If an equinus contracture is seen throughout the complete knee range of motion, then a formal Achilles tendon lengthening is indicated.

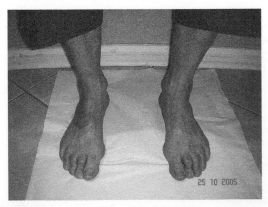

Fig. 1. Peek-a-boo heel sign.

Box 1
Etiologic classification for cavus foot
Brain
Tumor
Cerebral Palsy
Stroke
Spinal cord
Tumor
Poliomyelitis
Spinal dysraphism
Peripheral nervous system
Hereditary sensory motor neuropathy (eg, CMT)
Traumatic peripheral nerve injuries
Direct trauma to peripheral nerves
Muscle and tendon
Postsurgical clubfoot
Leg compartment syndrome
Duchenne's muscular dystrophy
Bone
Tarsal coalitions
Malunion of fractures (eg, talar neck)
Idiopathic

The hind foot should be assessed for sinus tarsi pain that may represent arthritis. Flexibility of the hind foot should be tested by the Coleman bloc test.[3] In this test, a 1 in block is placed under the lateral side of the foot, allowing the first metatarsal bone to drop. If the hind foot is flexible, and the hindfoot varus position is completely driven by a pronated forefoot, one will observe correction of the heel varus into valgus. If the heel alignment does not correct, a hind foot procedure must be added.

The forefoot must be examined for toe deformities including claw hallux, claw toes, callus, and pain under the metatarsal heads.

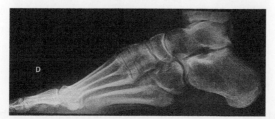

Fig. 2. Asymmetric right cavus foot secondary to spinal vascular malformation.

A complete neurologic examination must be performed including muscle strength testing.

RADIOGRAPHIC EVALUATION

Aminian and Sangeorzan[10] summarized the radiographic hallmarks of a cavus foot deformity as follows:

Increased calcaneal pitch (between line along the undersurface of the calcaneus and the floor; normal is 30°)

Increased angle of Meary (measured by the long axis of the talus and the first metatarsal; generally is 0°).

Increased Hibbs angle (between a line through the axis of the calcaneus and the first metatarsal; normal is less than 45°; cavus is near 90°)

A posterior fibula with a flat-topped talus. This artifactual appearance occurs because the lateral view is in fact oblique (**Fig. 3**).

A thorough radiographic analysis is mandatory to make conclusions about location of the apex of the deformity to choose the proper surgical technique for each case.

MEDICAL TREATMENT

The first approach must include identification of the etiology. In adults, nonprogressive deformity with mild symptoms is treated with symptomatic measures. For children, nonoperative treatment is indicated for nonsymptomatic cases and temporary symptomatic management for patients who cannot undergo for medical reasons. Progressive symptomatic deformity should be addressed surgically early in the course of the disease.

The most common symptomatic measures to treat cavovarus foot are inserts, shoe modifications, and physical therapy. These simple measures help most mild cavovarus foot deformities. The classic approach to making an insert is to unload points of excessive pressure with form-fitting arch supports using a longitudinal arch support. This device forces the patient to walk on the lateral side of the foot, blocking the ability to evert. In a more recent report, Chilvers and Manoli recommend dropping the head

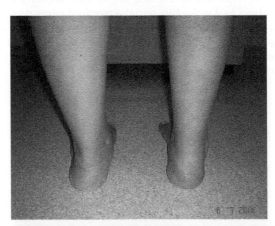

Fig. 3. Showing the typical flat talus on the lateral ankle radiograph and the other hallmarks of cavus foot.

of the plantar flexed first metatarsal into a depression in the orthotic and using a lateral forefoot post in an attempt to accommodate forefoot valgus in addition to lowering the arch support.[11] This alternative is an excellent idea; it provides good symptomatic relief, but it may create a thick orthosis that may not fit most shoes.

SURGICAL RECONSTRUCTION

Surgical management may be categorized broadly as soft tissue procedures, osteotomies, and arthrodesis. Most of these procedures tend to correct the static deformity of the cavus foot, but the dynamic deformity also must be addressed by tendon transpositions. The ultimate goal of surgery is to achieve a plantigrade foot with preservation of joints if possible.

Mild deformities require at least a plantar fascia release and dorsiflexion osteotomy of the first metatarsal (**Fig. 4**). For most of the cavus foot deformities that need surgery, some form of calcaneal osteotomy is also necessary. For evaluating how flexible the varus hind foot is, the Coleman block test is performed to decide if it is necessary to add a hind foot procedure. With a rigid hind foot varus, either a valgizing calcaneal osteotomy or a valgizing subtalar fusion (if subtalar arthritis present) will be needed. If the Coleman block test shows that the hind foot varus corrects completely, however, just a forefoot procedure will suffice (a first metatarsal dorsiflexion osteotomy) to correct the hind foot varus, a forefoot-driven hind foot varus. Although this test is very useful, the clinical assessment of hind foot and forefoot flexibility is also needed (**Fig. 5**).

The apex of the deformity must be identified to choose the correct surgical procedure for each case. For most cases, the main deformity is in the first metatarsal, which is why the dorsiflexion osteotomy should be performed in almost every case.

The apex of the deformity can be located in the hind foot and midfoot, and it also can be present in the lesser metatarsals as well as the first. A combination of deformities additionally can be present, and a careful radiographic analysis must be performed to classify the deformity.

Once the apex of the deformity is corrected, flexibility and tendon balance must be addressed as it was analyzed previously. This evaluation must take into consideration medial soft tissue release and lateral ankle ligament reconstruction.

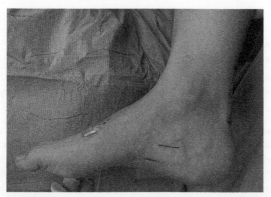

Fig. 4. Incisions for dorsiflexion osteotomy of first ray, plantar fascia release, and percutaneous lengthening of Achilles tendon.

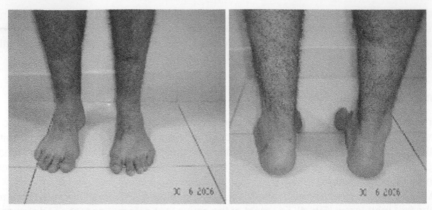

Fig. 5. Showing the clinical aspect of a long-term result of a left cavus foot that was corrected surgically with a dorsiflexion osteotomy of the first metatarsal, valgus calcaneal osteotomy, and plantar fascia release. The treated foot shows significant improvement when compared with the nonoperated contralateral side (the good foot). This surgery represents the most common combination of surgical procedures for mild cavus foot.

No correction will last over time if muscle power is not balanced. For most patients, a peroneus longus to brevis transfer is necessary to correct weak eversion and simultaneously weaken the plantarflexion of the first ray. For others, a weak anterior tibial tendon requires supplementation, such as a posterior tibialis tendon transfer to the dorsum of the foot.

In children, flexible deformities sometimes are solved only using soft tissue procedures. Fixed deformities require osteotomies, and arthritis requires arthrodesis in selected cases. In progressive deformities, it is particularly important to create a balanced foot, choosing the appropriate tendon transfers for each case. As a general rule, arthrodesis should be avoided in children younger than 8 years old, because this could result in growth arrest of more than 25% compared with the contralateral foot, which is thought to impair function.[8] An algorithm for hind foot, midfoot and forefoot corrections are presented (**Figs. 6** and **7**). The authors propose this step-by-step protocol to correct the deformity as a surgical guide and not as a recipe, because every deformity is unique. A summary of the surgical procedures is presented in **Box 2**.

CORRECTION OF STATIC DEFORMITY
Surgical Procedures

Soft tissue releases
In a cavovarus foot, contracted medial and plantar soft tissues are always present. For some deformities, a formal posteromedial release is required.

Plantar fascia release Every cavus foot needs a plantar fascia release, and this is usually the first procedure that most surgeons perform as part of the correction.

The authors perform a longitudinal incision 3 cm long between the plantar and the dorsal skin directly over the insertion of the plantar fascia. The fat tissue is retracted plantarwards below the abductor hallucis, and the plantar fascia is cut completely from medial to lateral using scissors.[12] In severe cavus feet, the abductor hallucis fascia also is contracted, and it can be released through this same approach.

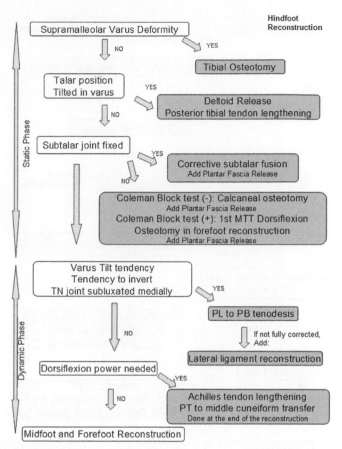

Fig. 6. Shows the algorithm for hind foot reconstruction. In the left side, the diagram shows the clinical situation that has to be evaluated. In the right side of the diagram, shaded in gray, appears the suggested surgical procedure.

Achilles tendon lengthening Some form of lengthening of the Achilles tendon is typically necessary. For most patients, the authors perform a percutaneous lengthening. Occasionally a gastrocnemius recession (slide) or a formal open Achilles tendon lengthening is required. A gastrocnemius recession is indicated if the gastrocnemius component alone is tight in the Silfverskiöld test. Excessive lengthening should be avoided to prevent an increase in cavus foot or the creation of a calcaneus gait with weak plantar flexion that also can result in ankle impingement.[13]

Other soft tissue procedures include medial soft tissue release of the ankle with respect to the deltoid ligament or posterior tibial tendon. Lateral ligament reconstruction with tendon autograft such as gracilis, plantaris or tendon allograft may be required.

Osteotomies
Supramalleolar osteotomies Cavovarus deformities may include supramalleolar deformities, where a supramalleolar varus deformity may be present. It is not known what extent of varus or valgus deformity will create arthritis in the ankle. Over 10°, in angular deformity in any plane will change the contact area in the ankle joint.[14]

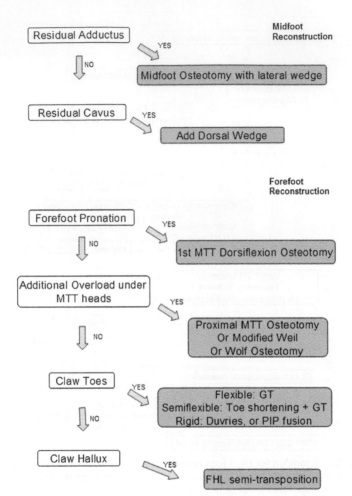

Fig. 7. Shows the algorithm for midfoot and forefoot reconstruction. In the left side, the diagram shows the clinical situation that has to be evaluated. In the right side of the diagram, shaded in gray, appears the suggested surgical procedure.

The association between a cavovarus foot and heel varus with ankle instability is known. This association, a common finding in cavovarus feet, can lead to degenerative arthritis.[15]

Significant varus alignment located at the distal tibia or at the ankle joint should be addressed, especially if early signs of osteoarthritis are present. The utility of osteotomies correcting varus malalignment in the setting of osteoarthritis at the ankle joint has been described with good results.[15,16] Takakura has shown good results using supramalleolar medial opening wedge osteotomies for varus ankle arthrosis.[17,18] The authors recommend lateral closing wedge osteotomies, to avoid using bone grafts, achieve immediate bone stability, and avoid increase soft tissue tension, as has been shown by Harstall.[16]

The authors currently perform supramalleolar lateral closing wedge osteotomies for varus deformities located at the ankle or distal tibia level. The osteotomy is performed 3 cm above the ankle joint, from the lateral side, considering the fibula and the tibia as

Box 2
Surgical procedures for cavus foot
Static deformities
Soft tissue procedures
Plantar fascia release
Percutaneous lengthening of Achilles tendon (if 90° are not reached with knee extended).
Osteotomies
Hindfoot fixed : "Z" calcaneal osteotomy
First metatarsal dorsiflexion osteotomy
Midfoot osteotomy: if apex of deformity is there and is severe
Arthrodesis
Double arthrodesis (subtalar and talonavicular joints)
Other procedures:
Medial soft tissue release of the ankle
Lateral ankle ligament reconstruction
Ankle arthroplasty
Dynamic deformities
Peroneous longus to brevis
Transfer of posterior tibialis to lateral cuneiform
Hammer toe correction
Soft tissue release
Resection arthroplasty or proximal interphalangeal (PIP) arthrodesis
G–T tendon transfer

a single bone, using the medial tibial cortex as a hinge. The authors do not add displacement to the osteotomy as recommended to realign the weight-bearing axis, because they want to keep the weight-bearing axis displaced to the lateral side of the joint, to load healthier cartilage and therefore decrease symptoms of ankle arthritis if present. As a general rule, the authors consider that 1 mm of lateral wedge will correct 1.2° at the ankle joint, and it will displace the weight -bearing point of the calcaneus 1.8 mm to the lateral side (Cristian Ortiz, MD, personal communication, 2008). The authors routinely fix the osteotomy with a small fragment plate on the fibula and on the tibia.

First metatarsal osteotomy As has been described by Manoli,[14] every subtle cavus foot needs a first metatarsal osteotomy, because plantar flexion of the first ray is always present.

The technique is very simple and is performed with a 3 cm longitudinal incision over the first metatarsal, and a perpendicular proximal cut is done 1 cm distal to the joint, perpendicular to the axis of the hind foot. The distal cut is done perpendicular to the axis of the first metatarsal close to 15°.[17] Usually a 4 mm to 5 mm wedge is removed, and the osteotomy is fixed with a 2.7 mm plate.

Another more stable technique has been reported by Hinterman,[7] in which the removed wedge is more parallel to the ground, making the osteotomy more stable (**Fig. 8**). The elevation obtained with this technique is twice as much, in millimeters,

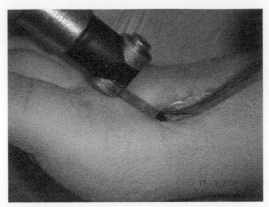

Fig. 8. Shows direction of the saw parallel to the plantar aspect of the foot to perform the osteotomy and remove the wedge.

as the base of the wedge removed (Cristian Ortiz, MD, personal communication, 2008). The wedge is usually between 4 mm and 6 mm, thus elevating the metatarsal between 8 mm and 12 mm. This is the authors' preferred way of performing the osteotomy, and fixation is achieved with two 2.0 mm screws from dorsal to plantar (**Fig. 9**).

Calcaneal osteotomies (Dwyer, Z osteotomy) With only rare exception, a calcaneal osteotomy is performed in addition to the first metatarsal osteotomy to correct rigid hindfoot varus (determined with a Coleman test). This has been the authors' experience, because most cavovarus feet already present to them with a fixed hindfoot deformity.

In the classic Dwyer osteotomy,[19] the technique is performed with an oblique incision below the peroneal tendons. If peroneal tendon transfer or lateral ankle ligament reconstruction is necessary, the incision can be extended proximally along the peroneal tendons. The sural nerve should be protected, retracting it superiorly or inferiorly as needed. The periosteum must be released widely to be able to remove the wedge, and an oscillating saw must be used. Fixation can be obtained with two 6.5 mm or 7.0 mm cannulated screws (**Fig. 10**).

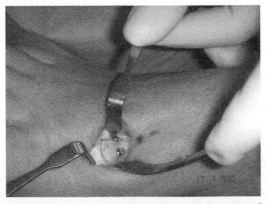

Fig. 9. Shows fixation with two 2.7 mm screws. **Fig. 8** shows direction of the osteotomy and position of the screws in a postoperative radiograph and a calcaneal osteotomy.

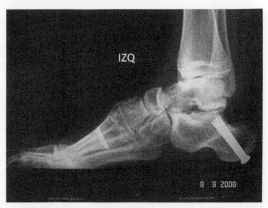

Fig. 10. Shows a lateral radiograph of the foot with a dorsiflexion osteotomy of the first ray a lateral sliding closing wedge osteotomy of the calcaneus.

The classic Dwyer osteotomy is very popular, but complete correction is obtained just in mild deformities. A lateral sliding calcaneal osteotomy is usually preferable for most cases.[13] A lateralizing calcaneal osteotomy will realign the hind foot varus during heel strike and will lateralize the moment arm of the Achilles tendon during toe off.

A triple correction calcaneal osteotomy can be performed when doing a lateral sliding calcaneal osteotomy, while removing a wedge and at the same time moving the calcaneal tuberosity proximal to decrease the calcaneal pitch. This correction may increase an existing ankle impingement, but it is a very powerful osteotomy correcting multiplanar deformities.

The L osteotomy described by Pisani and modified in a Z by Hintermann allows even more effective correction than the lateralizing closing wedge osteotomy for realignment of severe hind foot varus.[20]

For this osteotomy, a Homman retractor is placed over the top of the calcaneus behind the posterior facet, and a vertical cut is made. A longer horizontal cut is made at a right angle from this point. Another retractor is placed in the inferior corner of the calcaneus, and the second vertical cut is performed (see **Fig. 10**). At this point, a lateral based wedge is taken out, and lateral translation is obtained. In severe deformities, two vertical wedges can be removed to further correct sagittal deformity. Because this osteotomy is more proximal than the Dwyer, the correction of the tuberosity is more effective. This Z calcaneal osteotomy has become the authors' preferred osteotomy to correct hind foot in rigid cavus foot, because it is extremely powerful, offering a big contact surface for easy and stable fixation with two 7.0 cannulated screws.

Midfoot osteotomies: Cole, Japas, Akron Most surgeons try to avoid midfoot osteotomies, because they are hard to fix without crossing the adjacent joints and have a higher rate of wound complications than the other corrective procedures for cavus foot. Despite these difficulties however, they are absolutely necessary when the midfoot is the apex of deformity. Some authors try to replace the midfoot osteotomy with multiple metatarsal osteotomies, however, because the apex of the deformity is commonly more posterior, the end result is a foot with a Z deformity (**Fig. 11**).

These osteotomies are performed with one midline incision or two (medial and lateral) incisions and require removing a dorsal wedge to correct the cavus deformity and occasionally a biplanar component, adding a lateral wedge to correct adductus.

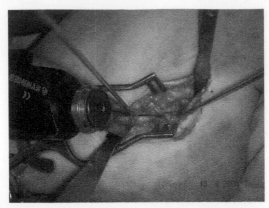

Fig. 11. Shows second and inferior vertical cut to complete the "Z" calcaneal osteotomy.

The osteotomy level can be performed at the tarsometatarsal joints (Jahss osteotomy)[21] or at the naviculocuneiform level (Cole and Japas[6]). The Akron dome osteotomy corrects the deformity were the apex frequently is located.[22] For most patients, the authors prefer an Akron type of osteotomy that crosses from the cuboid to the medial cuneiform and fix it with cannulated 3.5 screws. All midfoot osteotomies require internal fixation to decrease the high rates of nonunions and malunions, arthritis, shortening, and metatarsalgia that are reported in literature. For these reasons, midfoot osteotomies are not very popular for most surgeons performing cavus foot surgeries.

Arthrodesis

Although arthrodesis to correct deformities is considered by most surgeons as a failure, it remains a powerful technique to correct neurologic, recurrent, rigid, or severe deformities, especially in low-demand patients.

The concern that in the long term a triple arthrodesis will inevitably result in painful ankle arthritis does not seem to be true for all patients, specifically in those who have neurologic disorders, secondary to their minimal demand.

Several techniques have been recommended for hind foot arthrodesis, and all of them require rigid fixation to decrease the rate of nonunion that most commonly occurs at the talonavicular joint.

For a classic triple arthrodesis, there has been a trend toward leaving the calcaneo–cuboid (c-c) joint without fusing it, using as an argument that it commonly does not hurt and it is seldom arthritic. Fusing the c-c joint will decrease the accommodating capacity of the hind foot further when walking on uneven ground. When doing a triple arthrodesis, the authors are fusing just the subtalar and talonavicular joints, with similar results to the triple fusion (Cristian Ortiz, MD, personal communication, 2008).

The ultimate purpose of surgery is to create a plantigrade foot, and it must be obtained even using an arthrodesis in selected cases.

Ankle arthritis is commonly present in end-stage cavovarus foot deformities caused by the varus and the externally rotated tibia that produce an anterolateral extrusion of the talus resulting in ankle instability and arthritis. Although ankle arthrodesis remains the gold standard solution for most painful ankle arthritis, ankle replacement with the new-generation prosthesis has become more popular and is making orthopedic surgeons consider it as the best solution for some of these patients. Ankle replacement is the authors' method of choice to reconstruct cavovarus feet with end-stage ankle arthritis, and it is an option that has to be evaluated in a well-performed protocol to correct the whole forefoot and hind foot deformity.

CORRECTION OF DYNAMIC DEFORMITY (TENDON TRANSFERS)

Most of the time, tendon transfers are performed in conjunction with bony correction and soft tissue releases. The authors prefer to perform these transfers after the static deformities have been corrected. Different options have been described including:

Peroneus longus to brevis
Posterior tibial tendon to dorsum of the foot
Anterior tibial tendon to the middle of the foot
Extensor hallucis longus to neck of first metatarsal (Jones procedure)
Girdlestone Taylor transfer for hammer toe

Generally, specific requirements must be met for tendon transfers to be successful:

The tendon to be transferred should have similar strength (at least M4).
The tendon should be inserted close to the tendon to be replaced and routed without angulation.
There should be flexibility of the joints involved with the tendon transfer.
Fixation of the tendon should be to the bone directly or indirectly using another tendon.
Agonists are preferable to antagonists.
Tension should be half of the tendon excursion, although if there is any doubt, the authors prefer to leave it with a little bit more of tension.

These ideal criteria are not always and fully present; however, that should not prevent one from performing the tendon transfer. In these cases, the authors obtain a tenodesis effect, which is superior to a steppage gait.

Tendon transfers should be done after fixed deformities are corrected to achieve the appropriate tension of the tendon transferred.

Tendon transfers in cavus foot do not differ from other indications of tendon transfers, but incisions must be planned carefully especially when several incisions and osteotomies are performed at the same time. The approach may vary if the authors transfer the posterior tibial tendon to the middle cuneiform, the lateral, or even the cuboid if necessary.

Some controversy remains as to whether performing tendon transfers and osteotomies early are able to avoid triple arthrodesis in the future.[13] As a general rule, the authors prefer to indicate surgery as soon as the patient begins with symptoms unresponsive to medical treatment. During surgery, static and dynamic deformities must be corrected to avoid recurrence.

In less severe deformities, specifically in young patients, to prevent progression, the anterior tibial tendon can be transferred laterally to the middle cuneiform. In addition, a posterior tibial tendon lengthening can be added.[23]

Some other soft tissue procedures include medial foot and ankle release in cases of severe cavovarus and reconstruction of the lateral ankle ligaments. When a lateral ankle ligament reconstruction is needed, harvesting local tissues should be avoided, and some kind of graft must be used. For this purpose, reconstruction with gracilis, semitendinous, or some kind of allograft have been suggested.[24]

Peroneus Longus to Brevis Transfer

The most commonly performed tendon transfer is the peroneus longus to brevis to decrease the plantar flexion force of the peroneus longus and to increase the eversion power of the brevis to correct flexible varus. The maximal advantage is achieved in younger patients. The transfer can be done distally over the cuboid using the same incision for the osteotomy of the calcaneus or proximally behind the distal fibula. The peroneus longus is pulled distally under maximal tension and then slightly released to be sutured to the brevis using at least four stitches with nonabsorbable zero sutures.

Posterior Tibial Tendon Transfer

The second most common tendon transfer that the authors perform is tibialis posterior to one of the cuneiform bones. The chosen cuneiform depends on where the deformity corrects better, and there is no general rule for all cases. This transfer is particularly necessary in CMT. This transfer decreases the varus moment of the heel and augments the weakened dorsiflexion power of the tibialis anterior.

Extensor Hallucis Longus to First Metatarsal

The cock up deformity of the great toe is produced by the plantar flexion of the first metatarsal secondary to the overpowered peroneus longus and plantar fascia and the excessive pull by the extensor hallucis longus that is attempting to compensate for the weak anterior tibialis.

For children, the Jones transfer of the extensor hallucis longus to the neck of the first metatarsal is enough most of the time. For adults, the dorsiflexion osteotomy of the first metatarsal corrects most of the deformity; however, if not sufficient, a flexor to extensor tendon transfer must be added, in a similar technique as the Girdlestone Taylor transfer for the lesser toes. It is especially useful when there is a cock up deformity of the great toe and flexible plantar flexion of the first metatarsal. The authors have tried transferring half of the flexor hallucis longus to the proximal phalanx with goods results. For most adults, this procedure alone is not enough to correct the plantar flexion of the first ray, and an osteotomy must be performed. When done, if the flexor hallucis longus (FHL) was transferred completely, an interphalangeal fusion of the hallux must be performed.

Gilderstone Taylor Transfer

The transfer of the flexor digitorum longus to the dorsal aspect of the toe is useful for flexible deformities and is less predictable for the common rigid claw toes found in cavus foot. Most of the time, a resection arthroplasty or an interphalangeal fusion is added.

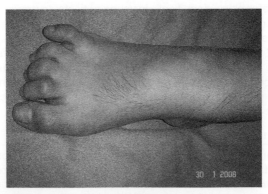

Fig. 12. Shows preoperative picture demonstrating claw toes.

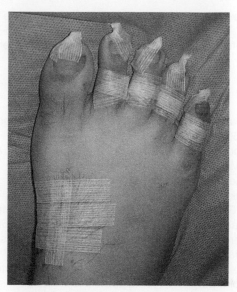

Fig. 13. Demonstrating correction of claw toes after resection arthroplasty lesser toes.

METATARSALGIA AND CLAW TOE CORRECTION

If prominent metatarsal heads are still evident after hind foot and midfoot procedures, a dorsiflexion osteotomy of the lesser metatarsals is needed. Several different techniques have been described to elevate the metatarsal heads, but the authors have found two recently reported techniques by Maceira[25] and Rippstein (Rippstein P, MD, personal communication, 2008) to be very useful.

Espinosa, Maceira, and Myerson[25] reported that a classic Weil osteotomy will not elevate the metatarsal heads, as it is needed for a cavus foot. A modified osteotomy is recommended with resection of a piece of the metatarsal with cuts perpendicular to the bone, achieving shortening and elevation in the axis of the bone. Rippstein reported his technique for elevation of lesser metatarsal heads by performing a proximal wedge resection with cuts parallel to the ground obtaining a stable fixation with screws. The claw toe correction is achieved best when the foot and ankle are balanced to choose the best techniques to avoid recurrence. For most patients, the authors begin with soft tissue balance with dorsal release of the metatarsophalangeal joints and plantar release of the flexor digitorum brevis and even flexor digitorum longus.

The claw toe correction is achieved best when the foot and ankle are balanced to choose the best techniques to avoid recurrence. For most patients, the authors begin with soft tissue balance with dorsal release of the metatarsophalangeal joints and plantar release of the flexor digitorum brevis and even flexor digitorum longus.

If this is not enough to obtain proper alignment, the authors perform a Du Vries resection arthroplasty of the proximal phalanx and fix it with percutaneous Kirschner wire (**Figs. 12–13**).

SUMMARY

Although the classical surgical options for reconstruction of cavovarus foot remain the basis for reconstruction surgery, new options and combination of procedures have become available and made early surgical reconstruction more likely.

Unfortunately, no evidence-based level one studies show the best way to reconstruct this deformity. This is why the authors propose this step-by-step protocol to correct cavovarus deformities as a surgical guide and not as a recipe, because every deformity is unique.

REFERENCES

1. Manoli AM, Graham B. The subtle cavus foot, the under pronator, a review. Foot Ankle Int 2005;26(3):256–63.
2. Brewerton D, Sandifer P, Sweetnam D. Idiopathic pes cavus. An investigation into its aetiology. Br Med J 1963;2:659–61.
3. Holmes J, Hansen SJ. Foot and ankle manifestations of charcot-marie-tooth disease. Foot Ankle 1993;14:476–86.
4. Nagai MK, Chan G, Guikke JT, et al. Prevalence of Charcot Marie tooth in patients who have bilateral cavovarus feet. J Pediatr Orthop 2006;26(4):438–43.
5. Mark R. Midffot and Forefoot issuees cavovarus foot: assessment and treatment issues. Foot Ankle Clin 2008;13(2):229–41.
6. Japas L. Surgical treatment of pes cavus by tarsal V-osteotomy. preliminary report. J Bone Joint Surg Am 1968;50:927–44.
7. Evans D. Relapsed club foot. J Bone Joint Surg Br 1961;43:722–33.
8. Lee M, Sucato D. Pediatric issues with cavovarus foot deformities. Foot Ankle Clin 2008;13:199–219.
9. Coleman SS, Chesnut WJ. A simple test for hindfoot flexibility in the cavovarus foot. Clin Orthop 1977;123:60–2.
10. Aminian A, Sangeorzan BJ. The anatomy of the cavus foot deformity. Foot Ankle Clin 2008;13(2):191–8.
11. Chilvers M, Manoli A II. The subtle cavus foot and association with ankle instability and lateral foot overload. Foot Ankle Clin 2008;13:315–24.
12. Steindler A. Operative treatment of pes cavus: stripping of the os calcis. Surg Gynecol Obstet 1917;24:612.
13. Krause F, Wing K, Alastair Y. Neuromuscular issues in cavovarus foot. Foot Ankle Clin 2008;13:243–58.
14. Swords M, Nemec S. Osteotomy for salvage of the arthritic ankle. Foot Ankle Clin 2007;12:1–13.
15. LaClair SM. Reconstruction of the varus ankle from soft-tissue procedure 14 with osteotomy through arthrodesis. Foot Ankle Clin 2007;12:153–76.
16. Harstall R, Lehmann O, Krause F, et al. Supramalleolar lateral closing wedge osteotomy for the treatment of varus ankle arhrosis. Foot Ankle Int 2007;28(5):542–8.
17. Takakura Y, Tanaka Y, Kumai T, et al. Low tibial osteotomy for osteoarthritis of the ankle: results of a new operation in 18 patients. J Bone Joint Surg 1995;77-A(1):50–4.
18. Myerson M. Cavus foot correction. In: Meyerson M, editor. Reconstructive foot and ankle surgery. Philadelphia: Elsevier; 2005. p. 153–68.
19. Dwyer F. Osteotomy of the calcaneum for pes cavus. J Bone Joint Surg Br 1959;41:80–6.
20. Pisani G. Osteotomia soototalamica di sottrazione laterale. In: Pisani G, editor. Tratato di chirugia del piede. Torino (Italy): edizioni Minerva Medica S.p.A; 1990. p. 297–8 [in Italian].
21. Jahss M. Tarsometatarsal truncated-wedge arthrodesis for pes cavus and equinovarus deformity of the fore part of the foot. J Bone Joint Surg Am 1980;62:713–22.

22. Wilcox PG, Weiner DS. The Akron midtarsal dome osteotomy in the treatment of rigid pes cavus: a preliminary review. J Pediatr Orthop 1985;5:333–8.
23. Klaue K. Hindfoot issues in the treatment of the cavovarus foot. Foot Ankle Clin 2008;13:221–7.
24. Hintermann B. Surgical tecniques. In: Total ankle arthroplasty. Wien (Austria): Springer Wien; 2005. p. 105–26.
25. Espinosa N, Maceira E, Myerson M. Current concepts review: Metatarsalgia. Foot Ankle Int 2008;29(8):871–9.

Reconstruction of Multiplanar Deformity of the Hindfoot and Midfoot with Internal Fixation Techniques

Thomas Dreher, MD, Sebastién Hagmann, MD, Wolfram Wenz, MD*

KEYWORDS

- Hindfoot reconstruction • Osteotomy • Arthrodesis
- K-wires • Internal fixation techniques • Cavovarus
- Charcot's foot • Planovalgus

Various complex multiplanar deformities of the foot in children and in adults need mid- and hindfoot reconstruction as an important step for the surgical correction (**Table 1**).

Many different neurologic and nonneurologic causes can be responsible for the deformity. The reconstruction strategies differ with regard to the possible underlying pathologies. It is therefore of greatest importance to identify all components and the pathogenesis, to understand the etiology of the deformity, and to distinguish between neurologic and nonneurologic pathologies.

It is common to combine different soft-tissue procedures ("balancing") and bony procedures ("correction") for the correction of multiplanar deformities (eg, talipes cavovarus in Charcot-Marie-Tooth disease [CMT].[1]) Exceptions are individual nonneurologic deformities such as idiopathic juvenile talipes planovalgus, tarsal coalition, Charcot's foot, and osteoarthritic deformities that do not require soft-tissue balancing.

PRINCIPLES OF HINDFOOT CORRECTION AND FIXATION
Hindfoot Osteotomies and Fusions

Joint fusions, osteotomies, or both are the basis for hindfoot reconstruction. To choose between articular (fusion) and extra-articular (osteotomy) correction, the level of the deformity and the degree of joint hypermobility, stiffness, or osteoarthritis should be examined and considered in the preoperative planning. Furthermore, different underlying pathologies require different approaches. For example, due to

Division of Pediatric Orthopaedics and Foot Surgery, Orthopaedic Department, University of Heidelberg, Schlierbacher Landstrasse 200a, Heidelberg 69118, Germany
* Corresponding author.
E-mail address: wolfram.wenz@ok.uni-heidelberg.de (W. Wenz).

Foot Ankle Clin N Am 14 (2009) 489–531
doi:10.1016/j.fcl.2009.06.001
1083-7515/09/$ – see front matter © 2009 Elsevier Inc. All rights reserved.

foot.theclinics.com

Table 1		
Foot deformities needing correction in the mid- and hindfoot		
Deformity	**Components**	**Etiology**
Equinus	Limited dorsiflexion in ankle	Idiopathic Secondary (eg, gastrocnemius hemangioma) Neurogenic (eg, CP, TBI, brain tumors, ICB, multiple sclerosis) Posttraumatic (eg, compartment syndrome) Compensatory (eg, leg length discrepancy)
Clubfoot	Hindfoot equinus Hindfoot varus Cavus Adductus Forefoot supination	Congenital, residual Neurogenic (eg, AMC, MMC, CP, TBI, apoplexy, myotonic dystrophia, spastic spinal paralysis, tethered cord, diastematomyelia, paraplegia) Posttraumatic (eg, compartment syndrome)
Cavovarus	(Hindfoot equinus) Drop foot Hindfoot varus Cavus Forefoot pronation Claw toes	Charcot-Marie-Tooth disease Other neurogenic causes (eg, CP, spastic spinal paralysis, myotonic dystrophy [Curschmann-Batten-Steinert syndrome], spinal muscular atrophy [Kugelberg-Welander syndrome]) Idiopathic
Planovalgus	Hindfoot equinus Hindfoot valgus Planus Abductus (Hallux valgus)	Congenital (talus verticalis) Idiopathic (juvenile, AAFD) Secondary (eg, coalition) Neurogenic (eg, CP, AMC, MMC, TBI, apoplexy, spastic spinal paralysis, tethered cord, ataxia) Syndrome associated (eg, Down syndrome)
Charcot's foot	(Hindfoot equinus) various, depending on type (see text)	Neuropathic (eg, diabetes, alcohol, toxic, polyneuropathy) Idiopathic
Calcaneal foot	Often concomitant deformities	Iatrogenic (eg, after TAL) Neurogenic (eg, MMC, tethered cord, CP) Congenital
Osteoarthritis	With or without accompanying hindfoot deformities	Idiopathic Secondary (eg, posttraumatic, infection)

Abbreviations: AAFD, adult acquired flatfoot deformity; AMC, arthrogryposis multiplex congenita; CP, cerebral palsy; ICB, intracranial bleeding; MMC, myelomeningocele; TAL, Achilles tendon lengthening; TBI, traumatic brain injury.

the tendency for recurrence of spastic planovalgus deformity in cerebral palsy following extra-articular correction, stabilization by way of joint fusion is considered in many cases. On the other hand, a juvenile idiopathic planovalgus foot is preferentially treated by extra-articular procedures.

Osteotomies

Table 2 gives an overview of the most important corrective osteotomies in the hindfoot, ignoring all forefoot osteotomies and special osteotomies used in combination with an external fixation system (tubes or frames).

Osteotomies can be performed with an oscillating bone saw, a Gigli's wire saw, a chisel, or an osteotome. The choice of technique depends on the surgeon's preference. Independent of the chosen technique, cooling during the sawing process reduces the prevalence of heat necrosis.[8] A minimum distance to the joint surface or the growth plate in children should be maintained to avoid injury or devascularization.

Joint fusions

Table 3 shows an overview of the key joint fusion procedures for the correction of multiplanar deformities of the hind- and midfoot.

There are three principles of fusion: resection, additive, and sparing. A severe midfoot cavus, for example, should be treated by resecting a dorsal-based wedge from Chopart's joint. Fusions can also be done as an additive procedure (eg, the calcaneocuboid distraction-arthrodesis). After removal of the cartilage, a bony wedge is inserted to lengthen the lateral border of the foot.

Sparing and additive fusions should be performed with a shaped chisel, taking into consideration the concave and convex site of the joint. Resection fusions can be done with the oscillating bone saw after preoperative planning.

Bone Fixation After Osteotomy or Arthrodesis

The surgeon may choose between different modalities for fixation after corrective osteotomy or joint fusion: plates, screws, Kirschner wires (K-wires), staples, or nails (**Table 4**).

Table 2
Key osteotomies for mid- and hindfoot correction

Osteotomy and Surgical Technique	Indication
Supramalleolar osteotomy[59,60] (derotation, varisation, valgisation, extension, flexion)	Increased/decreased tibial torsion after foot correction Varus/valgus deformity of the ankle Tibial flexion or extension deformity
Dwyer osteotomy[27] (lateral-based calcaneal wedge osteotomy)	Hindfoot varus Stability of subtalar and Chopart's joint
Gleich osteotomy[2,3] (medial calcaneal sliding osteotomy)	Hindfoot valgus Residual hindfoot valgus after Evans procedure or calcaneocuboid distraction-arthrodesis
Evans osteotomy[4,5] (lengthening osteotomy of the calcaneal neck)	Planovalgus foot Skew foot Stability of Chopart's or subtalar joint
Cole osteotomy[6] (dorsal-based wedge osteotomy in the midfoot)	Cavus foot, apex distally to Chopart's joint Stability of Chopart's joint
McHale osteotomy[7] (open wedge osteotomy of the medial cuneiform bone and closed wedge of the cuboid bone)	Structural fore/midfoot adductus Skew foot

Table 3
Key joint fusions for mid- and hindfoot correction

Arthrodesis and Surgical Technique	Indication
Ankle arthrodesis (tibiotalar/ tibiocalcaneal fusion)	Charcot's foot Severe varus/valgus instability Osteoarthritis
Subtalar fusion (lateral or medial open or closed wedge)	Hindfoot varus/valgus with instability Severe bony fixed varus/valgus Osteoarthritis
Triple arthrodesis (Chopart's and subtalar joint fusion)	Charcot's foot Severe planovalgus Cavovarus with severe hindfoot varus Severe clubfoot (residual)
Lambrinudi procedure[9] (triple fusion and subtalar ventral-based wedge resection)	Ventral talus impingement at the tibia (Bony) fixed hindfoot equinus
Inverse Lambrinudi[10] (additive triple fusion and subtalar dorsal-based wedge resection)	Severe calcaneal foot
Grice procedure[11]	Paralytic planovalgus foot (young children)
Chopart's arthrodesis	Clubfoot Cavovarus foot Charcot's foot
Calcaneocuboid distraction-fusion	Planovalgus foot
Naviculocuneiform arthrodesis	Instability

The authors prefer transcutaneous K-wires for the fixation for most of the primary fusions and osteotomies. K-wires are inexpensive and can be easily removed during and after surgery. With the transcutaneous technique, the wires remain in the foot only for the first period of bone healing (adults: 6 weeks; children: 4 weeks) and are then removed in the postoperative outpatient treatment with pliers under local anesthesia or sedation (children). K-wires are considered for all children, adolescents, and adults up to age 60 years. Exceptions exist for smokers, patients who have concomitant diabetic foot syndrome, vascular problems, and patients who have nonunion in their history. For those patients and all adults older than 60 years, cannulated screws, compression screws, and angle-stable locking plates are recommended for fixation.

The reconstruction philosophies of three typical foot deformities (cavovarus, adult acquired flatfoot deformity (AAFD) foot, and the diabetic Charcot's foot) are treated in the following sections. On the basis of these deformities, the principles of hindfoot reconstruction using different internal fixation systems can be elaborated.

CHARCOT-MARIE-TOOTH DISEASE AND CAVOVARUS FOOT
Charcot-Marie-Tooth Disease

CMT is also known as hereditary motor and sensory neuropathy or peroneal muscular atrophy. It is the most common inherited disorder of the peripheral nervous system and affects approximately 36 in 100,000 people.[12–14] It is caused by mutations inducing the loss or dysfunction of essential molecules necessary for nerve physiology,[14–17] which leads to loss of muscle bulk and touch sensation in the feet and legs. CMT may also affect the upper extremities. The muscular atrophy follows a certain chronology, causing muscular imbalance and leading to foot deformity. The most common foot

Table 4
Important internal fixation techniques for mid- and hindfoot reconstruction

Internal Fixation	Cost	Advantages and Disadvantages	Indication Criteria
K-wires	Low	Inexpensive Easy to use Temporary (easy to remove) Transcutaneous infection	All deformities in children, adolescents, and adults ≤60 y old Not indicated in Charcot's foot
Staples	Low-mid	Considerd only as an additional fixation system for hind-foot correction (eg. + K-wires) Costly to explant	Forefoot osteotomies Additive fixation, combined with K-wires
(Compression) cannulated screws	Mid-high	More stable than wires Compression is possible More expensive Costly to implant Costly to explant	Possible in all deformities of adolescents and adults Nonunions Smokers Reduced bone quality Charcot's foot
Angle-stable locking plates	High	More stable than screws Polyaxial fixation is possible More expensive Costly to implant Costly to explant	Ankle fusion Long-distance fusions Nonfusions Smokers Reduced bone quality Charcot's foot
Nails	High	†	Ankle/pantalar fusion Nonunions

† See chapters in this issue regarding hind-foot nails.

deformity in CMT patients is the cavovarus foot accompanied by claw toes. Furthermore, CMT is the most common cause of cavovarus feet: of 148 children, 116 (78%; mean age, 10 years; range, 3–18 years) who had bilateral cavovarus deformity had CMT.[15] Usually, the first clinical manifestations begin in late childhood or early adulthood, but symptom onset and progression of CMT may vary among patients.

Anatomy and Pathomechanics of Cavovarus Foot

The cavovarus foot in patients who have CMT is characterized by drop foot, hindfoot varus (subtalar), forefoot equinus (cavus), plantar flexion of the first metatarsal, and concomitant claw toes.[18] Furthermore, a limited dorsiflexion of the ankle (hindfoot equinus, dorsal impingement) can be found in many patients who have CMT and cavovarus foot.

The drop foot component can be attributed to the weak anterior tibial muscle. The imbalance between the strong peroneus longus muscle and weak anterior tibialis muscle[19] leads to increased plantarflexion of the first metatarsal and therefore to pronation of the forefoot. In addition, the peroneus brevis muscle is weaker than the posterior tibialis muscle, leading to a medial shift of Chopart's joint, and locks the subtalar joint in varus. The increased pronation of the forefoot aggravates this hindfoot varus during standing or during the stance phase of walking. The imbalance between the intrinsic and extrinsic foot muscles causes claw toe deformities. To compensate for the decreased dorsiflexion power of the anterior tibial muscle, the long toe extensors are excessively activated (extensor substitution). This compensatory mechanism aggravates the claw toe deformity.

The typical clinical manifestations of a bilateral cavovarus foot in CMT are shown in **Fig. 1**.

Preoperatively, the presence of CMT should be elucidated. The combination of bilateral cavovarus, muscular atrophy in forearm or hands, typical neurologic findings (clinical, electromyography, and nerve conductive velocities),[20,21] and a positive family history for cavovarus foot is sufficient. When there is further doubt about the diagnosis, a DNA test can identify the typical mutation for CMT and is therefore proof of the diagnosis of the disease.[20,21]

For the planning of surgical treatment, standardized clinical examination (range of motion, muscle (power) tests, Coleman block test, **Fig. 2**) and radiographic and dynamic examinations (dynamic pedobarography and instrumented three-dimensional [3D] gait analysis with foot model) are performed. **Fig. 3** shows the typical radiologic manifestations of a bilateral cavovarus foot in CMT.

Dynamic pedobarography is an objective method used to measure the dynamic pressure distribution pattern of the foot during walking.[22]

For the motion analysis of the single segments and joints of the foot during stance and swing phase of the gait, 3D gait analysis with a special foot model (eg, the Heidelberg foot model[23]) is performed.

Philosophy of Surgical Treatment in Cavovarus Deformity

For the correction of cavovarus foot deformity and to improve function of the foot during walking, various soft-tissue and bony procedures have to be performed during surgery. **Table 5** shows the chronology of surgical procedures for cavovarus correction considered by the authors.

Tendon transfers are used for soft-tissue balancing as active transfers or tenodesis (if an active control of the muscle is not possible). Bony procedures are used to correct

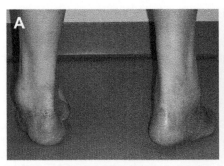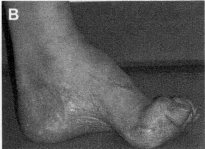

Fig. 1. Typical clinical manifestations of a cavovarus foot deformity in a 55-year-old man who has CMT. This deformity is characterized by different components: (A) hindfoot varus and equinus (hind- or forefoot) and forefoot pronation, and (B) cavus, flexion deformity of the first metatarsal, and claw toes.

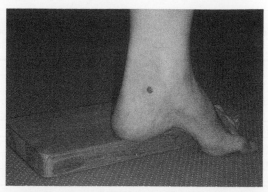

Fig. 2. Coleman block test for the determination of compensatory hindfoot varus as a consequence of fixed forefoot pronation. The patient's foot is placed on a 2- to 6-cm block, with the heel and lateral border of the foot bearing weight on the block. The first, second, and third metatarsals should hang freely into plantar flexion and pronation. When the heel is in neutral or slight valgus position, the hindfoot varus is caused by the increased pronation of the forefoot.

fixed deformities. Depending on the patient's age and bone quality and the extent of corrective means, K-wires, cannulated screws, or plates can be used to stabilize osteotomies and fusions. The authors commonly use K-wires for all children, adolescents, and adults up to age 60 years who have CMT. Exceptions exist for smokers, patients who have concomitant diabetic foot syndrome, and patients who have nonunion in their history. For those patients and all adults over the age of 60 years who have CMT, cannulated screws or plates are recommended for fixation. When a supramalleolar derotation or valgisation osteotomy is needed, osteosynthesis is done with K-wires in children and with an angle-stable locking plate for the distal tibia in adults.

The surgical correction starts with the plantar fascia release (Steindler procedure[24]). It may correct the cavus deformity in mildly involved cases. In most patients, the cavus component is fixed and only partially corrected by the Steindler procedure. Nevertheless, it should be performed in all cavovarus feet because later reposition of the foot after

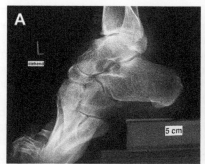
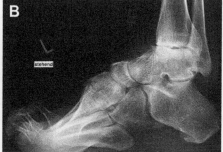

Fig. 3. Typical radiographs of a cavovarus foot in CMT. (*A*) Lateral view with concomitant Coleman block test. The ankle is nearly congruent. (*B*) Lateral view without block test. Typical findings: hindfoot varus (short calcaneus, open sinus tarsi sign, posterior rotation of the fibula, double dome sign [incongruency of the ankle]), cavus, flexion deformity of the first metatarsal.

Table 5
Chronology of surgical procedures for cavovarus correction in Charcot-Marie-Tooth disease

No.	Procedure	Necessity
1	Steindler[24]	■■■
2	T-SPOTT[26]	■■■
3	Bony reconstruction of the hindfoot (Chopart's fusion, triple fusion, and so forth)	▨▨
4	Fixation (K-wires, screws, plates)	■■■
5	Hindfoot equinus correction (Baumann[28], Strayer[29], TAL)	☐
6	Temporary ankle fixation (2.5 K-wire)	■■■
7	Modified Jones procedure[30,31]	▨▨
8	Extension osteotomy of the first metatarsal[25]	▨▨
9	Supramalleolar derotation/valgisation osteotomy[59,60]	☐
10	Tendon transfer completion	■■■
11	Claw toe correction of toes 2 through 5 (tenotomies, PIP-fusions)	■■■

Abbreviations: TAL, Achilles tendon lengthening; PIP, proximal interphalangeal joint; T-SPOTT, total split posterior tibial tendon transfer; ☐, necessary in a few cases; ▨▨, necessary in most of the cases; ■■■, necessary in all cases.

corrective osteotomy (Cole,[6] extension osteotomy of the first metatarsal[25]) or fusion (Chopart's arthrodesis) for cavus is easier. The advancement of the tendon transfers follows the Steindler procedure. The authors of this chapter successfully advanced and modified the typical surgical technique for posterior tibial tendon transfer[26] and labeled it as the total split posterior tendon transfer (T-SPOTT). The posterior tibial tendon is split into two halves and transferred through the interosseous membrane. One half is transferred medially to the anterior tibial tendon to augment the dorsiflexor moment arm; the other laterally augments the short peroneal tendon. The next step is bony correction of the cavus and hindfoot varus component. Extra-articular modalities (eg, Cole[6] and Dwyer[27] procedures) are indicated only in patients who have mild to moderate deformities and who have a stable Chopart's or subtalar joint. Because most of the patients show instability in Chopart's joint and the subtalar joint and often have recurrence of cavovarus following extra-articular bony correction, the authors recommend instead a Chopart's fusion with dorsal-based wedge resection for hindfoot reconstruction. In more severe cases or in cases that have limited ankle dorsiflexion due to ventral tibial impingement of the talus, a triple fusion or a Lambrinudi arthrodesis,[9] respectively, should be done.

The bony correction of the hindfoot is followed by an intraoperative clinical examination of the ankle range of motion and the foot tibial torsion. In the case of hindfoot equinus, a calf muscle lengthening (Baumann[28] or Strayer[29] procedure) or, in severe cases, an Achilles tendon lengthening (TAL) is needed. The hindfoot correction is followed by the modified Jones procedure[30,31] for claw toe correction, whereby the tendon of the extensor hallucis longus muscle is transferred to the first metatarsal through an osseous channel, and the interphalangeal joint is fused to avoid a hanging distal phalanx. In most cases, a complete correction of the plantar flexion deformity of the first metatarsal is not possible. An extension osteotomy of the first metatarsal[25] must be performed at the end of the surgery before the tendon transfers are sutured.

Rotational or varus deformities of the tibia are corrected by way of supramalleolar derotation/valgisation osteotomy. Then, at the end of the surgery, the tendon transfers

(T-SPOTT and extensor hallucis longus transfer) are sutured while the foot is held in a plantigrade position with adequate tension. Claw toes 2 through 5 should be treated afterward with a distal tenotomy of the flexors[32] and a proximal interphalangeal joint fusion depending of the extent of deformity. Another option is the flexor to extensor tendon transfer.[33]

Surgical Technique

In the beginning, the Steindler procedure is performed.[24] The origin of the plantar fascia at the calcaneus and the flexor digitorum brevis muscle is exposed as proximally as possible and released. The next step is the preparation of the posterior tibial tendon insertion at the navicular bone. The tendon is released as distal as possible. At the medial aspect of the lower leg, 3 to 4 cm proximal to the ankle, the tendon is pulled out (**Fig. 4**A) through another incision, split into two halves and tagged with No. 1 polyglycolid acid sutures (see **Fig. 4**B). The capsule of the talonavicular joint is incised and two Viernstein levers are inserted. More distally, the tendon of the anterior tibial muscle is exposed (see **Fig. 4**C). Both halves are transferred through the interosseous membrane to the extensor compartment (see **Fig. 4**D, E). Afterward, one half is transferred distally beneath the retinaculum extensorum through the tendon sheath of the anterior tibial tendon (see **Fig. 4**F). The preparation of the peroneal tendons through a lateral approach (4–5 cm, starting over the palpable peroneal tendons leading to the dorsum of the foot) is the next step. The sural nerve is exposed and tagged with a vessel loop. The tendon sheaths of the peroneal tendons are incised. The peroneus longus tendon is identified and tenotomized or lengthened (Z-lengthening). The peroneus brevis tendon is exposed and tagged. After the opening of the long toe extensors sheath, a corn forceps is driven proximally, and the second half of the posterior tibial tendon is grabbed and transferred distally (see **Fig. 4**G, H).

Afterward, cartilage from the talonavicular joint is removed with a shaped chisel medially (**Fig. 5**A). In cases of severe cavus deformity, a dorsal-based wedge is taken from Chopart's joint. An arthrodesis spreader is inserted to complete the cartilage removal. If wedge resection is not necessary, then the removal should be performed in a convex–concave manner for optimum fitting of the fusion later on. In adults, the authors consider milling of the bony surfaces with a 2.0 drill to achieve superior healing. Subsequently, at the lateral border of the foot, the extensor digitorum brevis origin is released from the anterior process of the calcaneus with a chisel to open the entrance to the calcaneocuboid joint (see **Fig. 5**B). The capsule is resected and two Viernstein levers are inserted, exposing the calcaneocuboid and the lateral aspect of the talonavicular joint (see **Fig. 5**C). The cartilage is removed with the shaped chisel in the same technique as medially (see **Fig. 5**D). When dorsal-based wedge resection is necessary, the osteotomy can also be done with an oscillating bone saw. All cartilage should then be removed (see **Fig. 5**E). When the hindfoot varus cannot be corrected sufficiently by Chopart's fusion or when there is severe instability in the subtalar joint, a triple fusion may be necessary. The lateral skin incision is extended, the sinus tarsi is exposed, and the capsule of the subtalar joint is incised. After insertion of the osteotomy spreader, all cartilage is removed from the joint surfaces. A lateral-based wedge in severe hindfoot varus can be taken with the oscillating bone saw. In the case of ventral talus impingement at the tibia or a fixed bony hindfoot equinus, a Lambrinudi arthrodesis[9] should be done by removing a ventral-based wedge from the subtalar joint with a bone saw.

The redression of the foot subsequently follows. It is important to dorsiflex the mid-/forefoot complex, whereas the hindfoot is fixed in slight valgus position. The lateral border is then supported with the thumb of one hand while the other fingers palpate

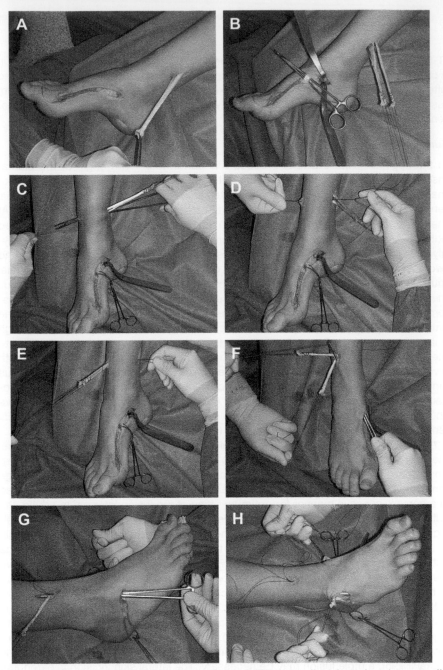

Fig. 4. T-SPOTT. (*A*) The posterior tibial tendon (PTT) is distally released and proximally pulled out with an Overholt clamp. (*B*) The tendon is split and both halves are tagged. Distally, the anterior tibial tendon (ATT) is exposed. (*C*) A slim corn forceps is driven through the interosseous membrane from medially to the anterior extensor compartment; a transfer loop thread is grabbed there and transferred medially. (*D*) The tag thread of the PTT halves are interlaced into the loop and the tendon halves are transferred anteriorly (*E*). (*F*) Subsequently, one PTT half is transferred through the tendon sheath of the ATT, while at the lateral border of the foot (*G*), the corn forceps is driven through the sheath of the extensor digitorum tendons to grasp the tag thread of the other PTT half. (*H*) Tendon transfer is complete.

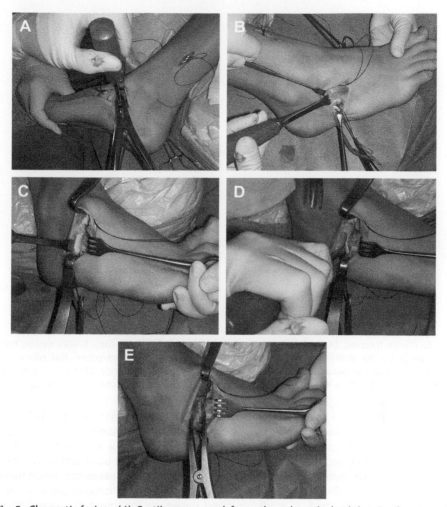

Fig. 5. Chopart's fusion. (*A*) Cartilage removal from the talonavicular joint. In the case of a severe cavus, a dorsal-based wedge is taken. (*B*) The origin of the extensor digitorum brevis muscle (anterior calcaneal processus) is released with a chisel for the approach to the calcaneocuboid joint. (*C, D*) Cartilage removal from the calcanealcuboid joint and lateral aspect of the talonavicular joint. (*E*) Arthrodesis spreader is inserted to remove all cartilage in the depth.

the calcaneocuboid joint. With the other hand, K-wires (2.5 mm for adults, 2.2 mm for children and adolescents) are inserted in the dorsum of the foot, approximately in the space between the fourth and fifth metatarsal, to fix the calcaneocuboid joint (**Fig. 6**A, B). At least two K-wires should be used for one joint. If a cannulated screw fixation is planned, then corresponding thinner K-wires are used and the screws are driven into the bone under guidance of the wires after a radiographic check. Accidental concomitant fixation of distal joints should be avoided when using screws. When there is need for long-distance fusion (eg, in concomitant diabetes, in osteoarthritis, or in the case of instability of the navicular-cuneiform and cuneiform-metatarsal joint 1), angle-stable locking plates should be used (see later section, "Outcome"). Afterward, the talonavicular joint is also fixed with two K-wires or screws (see **Fig. 6**C). In the case of

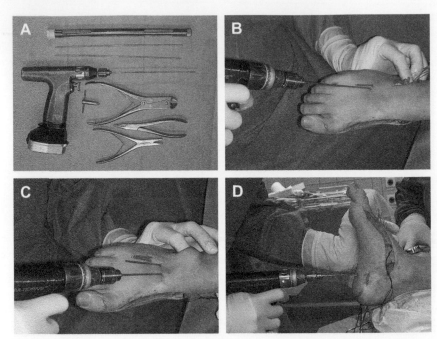

Fig. 6. K-wire fixation. (*A*) Tools for K-wire fixation technique (*from top*): K-wire depot; two K-wires (2.5 mm); drilling machine and key; wire cutter; long-nose pliers; flat pliers. (*B*) Transfixation of the calcaneocuboid joint with two K-wires. (*C*) Fixation of the talonavicular joint with another two K-wires. (*D*) Facultative K-wire fixation of subtalar and ankle joint.

additional triple or Lambrinudi[9] arthrodesis, two extra wires have to be inserted. These wires should be inserted from the lateral border of the foot and should run from posterior lateral plantar to anterior central dorsal, fixing the calcaneus and the talus. Alternatively, a crossing technique is possible. Radiographs should be obtained to check the position of the hardware. The ankle is now intraoperatively assessed. When there is limited ankle dorsiflexion due to calf muscle shortness, soft-tissue equinus correction should be performed. In mildly involved cases, an intramuscular recession is preferred (Baumann,[28] Strayer[29] procedures). In severe cases, TAL is indicated. After the foot is brought into plantigrade position, one K-wire can be driven through the calcaneus and the talus into the distal tibia for temporary fixation of the ankle (see **Fig. 6**D). The next step is the correction of the claw deformity of the first column. The modified Jones procedure[30,31] combines the transfer of the extensor hallucis longus to the first metatarsal and a fusion of the first interphalangeal joint. The tendon is distally tagged and released by an S-shaped skin incision. The distal part of the first metatarsal is exposed subperiostally (**Fig. 7**A). A 3.2-mm hole is drilled centrally in the first metatarsal. The tagged tendon of the extensor hallucis longus muscle is then transferred through the hole with a large needle sutured to itself (No. 1 Vicryl) at the end of the surgery (see **Fig. 7**B). Afterward, the interphalangeal joint is fused and fixed with two crossing K-wires (in children) or a compression screw (in adults). If the plantar flexion deformity of the first metatarsal cannot be corrected sufficiently by the modified Jones procedure (most of the cases), then an extension osteotomy[25] has to be performed. Therefore, the proximal part of the first metatarsal is exposed (see **Fig. 7**C) and a dorsal-based wedge is taken with the oscillating bone saw while the plantar corticalis is retained (see **Fig. 7**D). The osteotomy is then closed (see

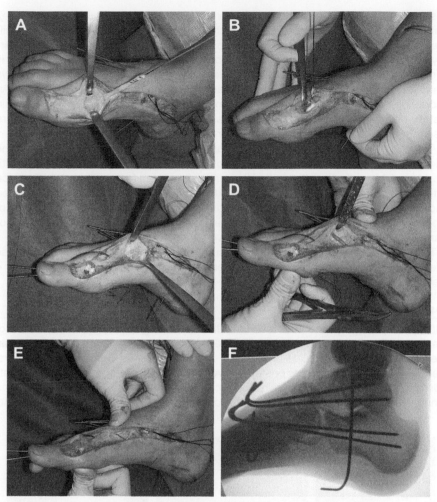

Fig. 7. Modified Jones procedure. (*A*) The extensor hallucis longus (EHL) tendon is tagged, released distally, and mobilized. The first metatarsal is subperiostally exposed. (*B*) After drilling a hole through the first metatarsal, the EHL tendon is transferred through the bone. Pulling the tag thread tests flexibility of the first metatarsal. Extension osteotomy is indicated when there is not enough correction of the flexion deformity. (*C*) The proximal part of the first metatarsal is exposed subperiostally. (*D*) A dorsal-based wedge is taken by oscillating bone saw, with the plantar corticalis intact. (*E*) Closing the osteotomy corrects the first tray. (*F*) Intraoperative radiograph after K-wire transfixation of Chopart' joint, the extension osteotomy of the first metatarsal, and the hindfoot.

Fig. 7E) and fixed with an angle-stable locking plate or with one or two crossing K-wires.

In some patients, there is malalignment of the tibia, especially in the transverse plane (external rotation deformity). It should be treated with a supramalleolar tibial osteotomy.[59,60] The approach at the medial tibia is extended proximally and the tibia is exposed subperiostally by insertion of Hohmann levers. Afterward, the corrective osteotomy can be performed. Isolated derotation osteotomy below 30° to 40° does not require an additional fibular osteotomy. When the needed correction exceeds this amount or there is need for a correction in the frontal or sagittal plane (very rare), a fibular osteotomy should be done before the tibial osteotomy. Osteosynthesis in children is done with four crossing K-wires (two from the medial malleolus, two from laterally). In adolescents and adults, distal tibial angle-stable locking plate fixation is considered. Before the osteotomy, the plate is already fixed with three to four screws distally. Then, the osteotomy height is marked and the plate is removed again. An oscillating bone saw is used for the osteotomy. Afterward, the plate is installed again distally and the correction is done (eg, internal rotation). The plate fixation pliers are inserted, and the three to four proximal screws are placed.

At the end of the surgery, the tendon transfers are sutured. At the lateral foot, the one half of the posterior tibial tendon is sutured to the peroneus brevis tendon with No.1 Vicryl. Medially, the other half of the tendon is sutured to the anterior tibial tendon with the same technique. Afterward, the extensor hallucis tendon is maximally pulled and sutured to itself. The last step is the correction of the claw toes with tenotomy of the flexor tendons,[32] proximal interphalangeal joint (PIP)-fusions, or flexor-to-extensor transfers.[33] **Fig. 7**F shows the intraoperative result after the correction.

The K-wires are shortened with the wire cutter and bent with flat pliers and long nose pliers (see **Fig. 6**A). They are maintained percutaneously for 6 weeks (in adults) or 4 weeks (in children) and can be easily removed after the required time period.

Postoperative Treatment

Initially after surgery, the foot is immobilized in a NightSplint™ (Darco, Raisting, Germany). The K-wire through the calcaneus, talus, and the tibia helps to maintain the neutral ankle position. Hilotherapie®, a cooling system (Hilotherm, Eisenharz, Germany) is installed to reduce postoperative swelling and hematoma. On the first postoperative day, radiographic examination is performed, the heel K-wire is removed, and a non-weight-bearing below-knee plaster cast in neutral ankle position with the heel

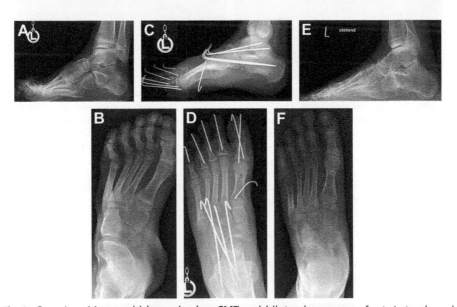

Fig. 8. Case 1: a 14-year-old boy who has CMT and bilateral cavovarus foot. Lateral- and anteroposterior (AP)-view radiographs taken preoperatively (*A, B*); at six weeks post surgery (*C, D*); and at 1-year postoperative follow-up (*E, F*).

held slightly in eversion is applied. If bony procedures were needed, then the plaster cast must not be burdened with load for 6 weeks (adults) or 4 weeks (children). After this time, another radiographic examination is done and the K-wires are removed with flat pliers under optional sedation. A removable weight-bearing plaster cast is then applied for another 6 weeks (adults) or 4 weeks (children). The physiotherapist starts to mobilize the ankle, applies special coordination training for the tendon transfers, and uses special force training. After the removal of the last plaster cast, an ankle-foot orthosis is used for about 6 months for walking long distances.

Outcome

Case 1

A 14-year-old boy presented with CMT disease. He suffered from bilateral cavovarus foot (**Fig. 8**A, B) with pain under the first and the fifth metatarsophalangeal joints, especially after walking long distances. He underwent surgery, with a combination of a Steindler procedure, a modified Jones procedure, a T-SPOTT, a Chopart's fusion, an extension osteotomy of the first metatarsal, and claw toe correction of toes 2 through 5. The fusions were fixed with K-wires appropriate for an adolescent. **Fig. 8**C and D show the 6-week postoperative outcome just before K-wire removal. The 1-year follow-up (see **Fig. 8**E, F) indicates a good radiologic result.

Case 2

Fig. 9 shows the preoperative and 1-year postoperative radiographs of a 26-year-old man who had CMT and bilateral cavovarus. For the correction of the right side,

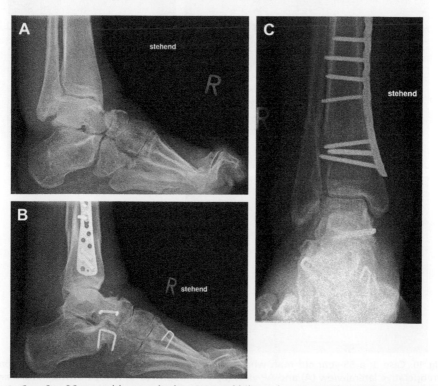

Fig. 9. Case 2: a 26-year-old man who has CMT and bilateral cavovarus foot. (*A*) Preoperative lateral-view radiograph. (*B, C*) Radiographs taken at 1-year postoperative follow-up.

a supramalleolar internal rotation osteotomy in addition to the standard surgical program (Steindler, T-SPOTT, modified Jones, Chopart's fusion, extension osteotomy of the first metatarsal, claw toe correction) was needed. The osteosynthesis was done with a distal tibial angle-stable locking plate.

Case 3

Fig. 10 shows the preoperative and 1-year postoperative clinical photographs and radiographs of a 55-year-old man who had CMT and bilateral symmetric cavovarus.

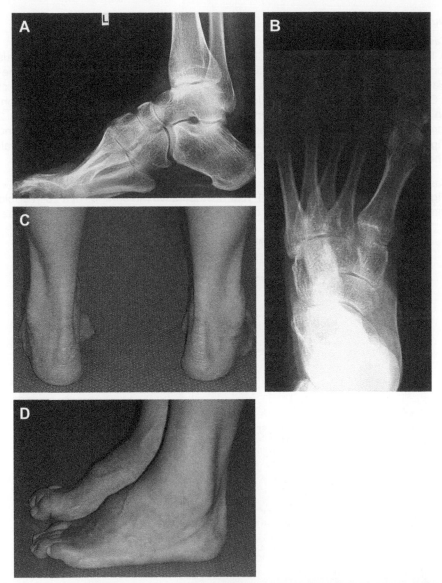

Fig. 10. Case 3: a 55-year-old man who has CMT and bilateral symmetric cavovarus foot. Preoperative lateral-view (*A*) and AP-view (*B*) radiographs. (*C–E*) Preoperative clinical manifestations. (*F, G*) Radiographs taken at 1-year postoperative follow-up. (*H–J*) Clinical outcome at 1-year postoperative follow-up.

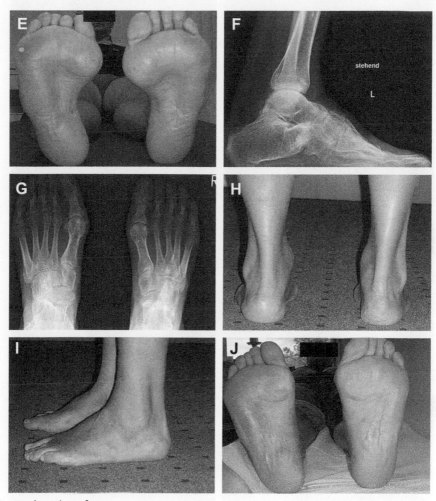

Fig. 10. (*continued*)

He was treated with a Steindler procedure, a modified Jones procedure, a T-SPOTT, Chopart's fusion, an extension osteotomy of the first metatarsal, and claw toe correction of toes 2 through 5. The patient suffered from no other diseases and had no history of nonfusion; therefore, the fusion fixation was done with K-wires. Intraoperative milling of the osteotomy surfaces was also performed, which was followed by problem-free bone healing.

Case 4
Fig. 11 shows the preoperative and 1-year postoperative clinical photographs and radiographs of a 55-year-old man who had CMT and bilateral symmetric cavovarus. The patient is a smoker and suffered from low-level diabetes. In addition to the standard surgical program (Steindler, T-SPOTT, modified Jones, Chopart's fusion, claw toe correction), the patient showed instability of the first metatarsocuneiform joint. The extension osteotomy of the first column was therefore done by a dorsal-based wedge resection fusion in the first metatarsocuneiform joint. The osteosynthesis was performed with a rearfoot plating system (RPS™); a 14-hole, long angle-stable

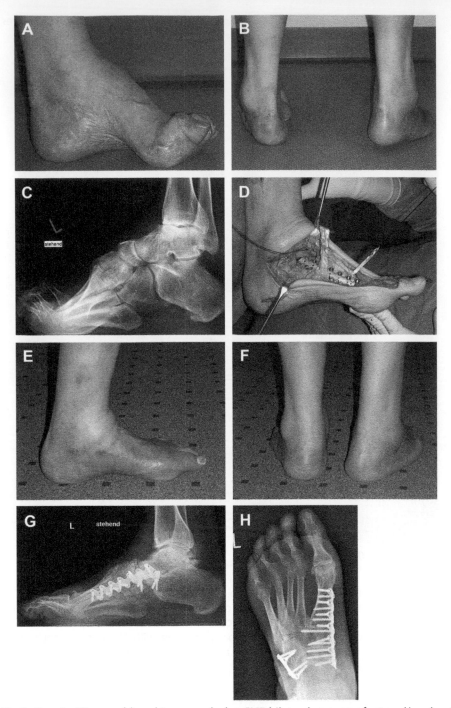

Fig. 11. Case 4: a 55-year-old smoking man who has CMT, bilateral cavovarus foot, and low-level diabetes. (*A, B*) Preoperative clinical manifestations. (*C*) Preoperatove lateral-view radiograph. (*D*) Intraoperative photograph. The angle-stable locking plate (14 holes, Darco) stabilizes the medial tray; the anterior tibial tendon is severely elongated after cavus correction; the extensor hallucis longus tendon is transferred to the first metatarsal. (*E, F*) One-year follow-up clinical outcome. (*G, H*) Radiographs taken at 1-year postoperative follow-up.

locking plate (Darco) at the medial border of the foot, including the talonavicular, the navicular-cuneiform and the first metatarsocuneiform joint (see **Fig. 11**D). The calcaneocuboid joint was fixed with a universal plating system 2.7 (UPS™); an extra 4-hole angle-stable locking plate (Darco).

Outcome Studies

Outcome studies presenting long-term results after complex foot reconstruction surgery in talipes cavovarus are rare. Most of the studies only report radiographic changes and neglect dynamic functional outcome. The authors consider foot-model analysis during instrumented 3D gait analysis an important tool for preoperative planning and outcome evaluation.

Significant improvements of the cavovarus deformity, as measured by radiographs (talus–first metatarsal angle, calcaneus–first metatarsal angle, and calcaneal pitch) and by pedobarography, were found by Chan and colleagues.[34] Furthermore, they recognized increased heel pressures after correction. Limitations of their study were the small number of patients (N = 9) and the lack of a 3D foot-model analysis. In another study, Azmaipairashvili and colleagues[35] evaluated 25 patients who had CMT and cavovarus foot. They too were able to show significant improvement in radiographic parameters after surgical correction. These investigators underlined the importance of graded treatment and considered soft-tissue procedures for young children and bony correction in older patients. Although this methodology should not be taken as a rule because the authors have seen a lot of recurrences following isolated soft-tissue correction, Azmaipairashvili and colleagues[35] further reported pain and arthritic signs after triple fusion and concluded that this procedure should be avoided if possible. This consideration is underlined by Wetmore and colleagues,[36] who found poor results after triple fusion in 50% of patients who had CMT. The authors use Chopart's fusion in most of the cases for bony hindfoot correction. The cavus and the varus component can be treated sufficiently with this method. Only a few feet need a triple or a Lambrinudi fusion. Extra-articular procedures (osteotomies) seem to have a higher recurrence rate. Prospective controlled clinical trials based on clinical, radiographic, and functional data: 3D foot-model analysis, dynamic pedobarography, e.g. EMED®(Novel GmbH, Munich, Germany) comparing different treatment strategies are needed for the optimization of cavovarus treatment in CMT.

RECONSTRUCTION OF PLANOVALGUS FOOT
The Planovalgus Foot: Etiology and Pathomechanics

The planovalgus foot is characterized by reduction or a loss of the normal medial longitudinal arch (pes planus) by hindfoot valgus/forefoot abduction and often occurs with concomitant hindfoot equinus. All these components can be flexible or rigid. The planovalgus foot can be found in 20% of the adult population, whereas about 80% of children have a flexible planovalgus foot. Different types of the planovalgus foot can be differentiated when considering etiology (**Table 6**).

Anatomic characteristics of the planovalgus foot include

Horizontalization of the calcaneus
Calcaneus in valgus and externally rotated relative to the talus
Verticalization of the talus, medial rotation of the talus
Subluxation of the talonavicular joint
Midfoot sag
Short lateral column in relation to the medial column
Forefoot abduction

Table 6
Types of planovalgus foot and indications for surgical treatment

Type	Indication	Surgical Techniques
Neurogenic (children ≥5–6 y)	Failed conservative treatment Moderate to severe deformity Pes valgus ab equino Midfoot break Instability Pain Secondary impairing of the gait due to deformity or instability (crouch gait, valgus knee, internal rotation gait)	PTL + Baumann or Strayer (TAL only in severe equinus) + (for mild and moderate deformity/stability in Chopart's joint): Evans/Grice ± Gleich (children) CCD-fusion ± Gleich (adolescents) or PTL + Baumann or Strayer (TAL only in severe equinus) + (for severe deformity/instability in Chopart's and subtalar joints): triple arthrodesis with lateral subtalar open wedge grafting
Neurogenic (adults)	Failed conservative treatment Moderate to severe deformity Pes valgus ab equino Midfoot break Instability Pain Secondary impairing of the gait due to deformity or Instability (crouch gait, valgus knee, internal rotation gait)	PTL + Baumann or Strayer or TAL + triple arthrodesis

Pediatric flatfoot (nonneurologic)	Only in symptomatic patients: Persistent pain Unsuccessful nonsurgical treatment Coalition	Mild: calcaneal-stop screw[37] or arthroereisis ± Baumann/Strayer/TAL Moderate to massive: Evans/Grice ± Gleich ± Baumann/Strayer/TAL Severe: triple arthrodesis ± Strayer/Baumann/TAL
AAFD	Stages 2 through 4 PTTD: 2A (hindfoot valgus with flexible forefoot varus) 2B (hindfoot valgus with forefoot abduction) 2C (flexible hindfoot valgus, fixed forefoot varus, first ray dorsiflexion) 3A (rigid hindfoot valgus) 3B (+ forefoot abduction) 4A (rigid hindfoot valgus + deltoid ligament insuffiency) 4B (rigid hindfoot valgus + ankle arthritis)	Gleich + Strayer/TAL ± FDL[38] Gleich + Evans + Strayer/TAL ± FDL Gleich, TMT joint fusion + FDL ± Strayer/TAL Triple fusion Triple fusion + CCD-fusion Triple fusion + ligament reconstruction Pantalar fusion

Abbreviations: CCD-fusion, calcaneocuboid distraction-fusion; FDL, flexor digitorum longus transfer to posterior tibial tendon;[39] PTL, peroneal tendon lengthening; PTTD, posterior tibial tendon dysfunction; TMT, tarsometatarsal.

In the pediatric population, flattening of the long arch, forefoot pronation, and hind-foot valgus are very common in infants and toddlers.[40] The severity of planovalgus is variable, and some ethnicities have a higher disposition. It seems that genetic deter-mination of ligament laxity plays a role in development of deformity. In most of the chil-dren, the planovalgus foot improves with age, mainly in the first decade.[41] Different investigators have reported only minimal influence of the muscular activity to the development, persistence, or deterioration of the pediatric planovalgus foot.[42,43] It is well known that a flexible planovalgus foot is more common in children who have shortened calf muscles or a shortened Achilles tendon.[41]

Most children who have flexible planovalgus foot are asymptomatic. The clinical examination is the most important tool used to distinguish between flexible and struc-tural (rigid) planovalgus. The flexible planovalgus foot corrects on heel rise, the arch restores, and the hindfoot inverts. A rigid planovalgus foot cannot be actively cor-rected on heel rise. Passive dorsiflexion of the first metatarsophalangeal joint leads to arch restoration in flexible flat foot (Jack test[44]). Symptomatic children commonly complain about tenderness around the talonavicular joint and early fatigue in the foot during longer walks. Secondary planovalgus deformities (eg, in coalition) should be separated from primary deformities.

The neurogenic planovalgus foot in children and adults can be caused by different etiologic disorders. The most common neurogenic disorders associated with plano-valgus foot are cerebral palsy (especially spastic diplegia/quadriplegia), spina bifida, apoplexy, and traumatic brain injury. The neurogenic planovalgus foot is the conse-quence of muscular imbalance caused by increased muscle tone of the peroneal muscles or weakness of the posterior tibial tendon. Furthermore, the planovalgus foot plays a role as a compensatory mechanism in equinus deformity (pes valgus ab equino). Patients who have toe walking may develop a planovalgus foot under the body load. In contrast to the nonneurogenic planovalgus foot in adults and chil-dren, surgical or nonsurgical treatment is considered for all feet, independent of clin-ical symptoms.

In the adult population, planovalgus deformity occurs in about 20%; most of these deformities are flexible and do not cause clinically relevant problems.[40] The most common cause of AAFD is posterior tibial tendon dysfunction (PTTD). Less often, the AAFD is idiopathic or is the consequence of diabetes (Charcot's foot, see later discus-sion) or neurogenic disorders. The etiology of PTTD comprises a large number of factors:

Flexible planovalgus foot
Traumatic (eg, ankle fracture, avulsion of the navicular bone, tendon dislocation, rupture, post injection, laceration)
Accessory navicular bone
Tarsal coalition
Inflammatory (eg, rheumatoid arthritis, spondylitis ankylosans, other types of arthritis)

Myerson[45] described a clinical staging for PTTD (**Box 1**).

Indications for Surgical Treatment in Planovalgus Foot

Indication criteria for surgical correction depend on the underlying pathology, the clin-ical symptoms, and the age of the patient (see **Table 6**).

Surgical Techniques

Calcaneal–stop screw technique
Indications This technique is very controversial.[37] Roth and colleagues[37] indicated this procedure for flexible idiopathic flatfoot in children. Alternatively, arthroereisis can be

> **Box 1**
> **Clinical staging of posterior tibial tendon dysfunction**
>
> Stage 1: No deformity, but pain over the posterior tibial tendon, with or without swelling
>
> Stage 2A: Flexible deformity with concomitant medial pain only[39]
>
> Stage 2B: Flexible deformity with concomitant lateral pain
>
> Stage 3: Rigid deformity
>
> Stage 4: Rigid deformity and concomitant changes at the ankle
>
> *Data from* Myerson MS. Adult acquired flatfoot deformity. J Bone Joint Surg 1996;78:780–90.

done with sinus tarsi implants.[46] It is important to consider postoperative pain, incomplete correction, need for early-removal surgery, and even structural bone changes[47] when planning this surgery.

Surgical technique A 1- to 1.5-cm skin incision is done at the lateral border of the foot over the sinus tarsi. The sinus fat is retracted and the dorsal aspect of the calcaneal neck is exposed in the sinus tarsi by the insertion of one small Hohmann lever. The heel is held in inversion, and a guiding K-wire is drilled into the calcaneus nearly perpendicular to the longitudinal axis of the calcaneal neck. Afterward, a radiographic check is done. If the wire is correctly placed, then a cannulated screw (6.5 mm) is inserted. The screw should have enough length so that the head of the screw is able to prevent subtalar motion into valgus by impinging at the lateral aspect of the talus (**Fig. 12**A, B).

Modified Evans procedure

A slightly S-shaped skin incision is done over the sinus tarsi.[4] The sural nerve and the peroneal tendons are identified and retracted. The neck of the calcaneus is subperiostally exposed by the insertion of the small Hohmann levers. The calcaneocuboid joint is then marked with a needle to ensure that the osteotomy is made at a sufficient

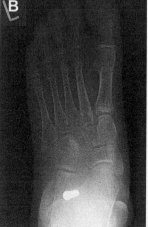
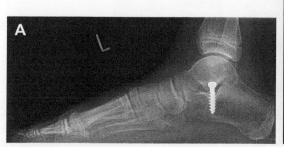

Fig. 12. Calcaneal–stop screw technique. (*A*) Lateral-view radiograph. (*B*) AP-view radiograph.

distance from this joint. Afterward, the osteotomy is done with an oscillating bone saw, perpendicular to the longitudinal axis of the calcaneus (**Fig. 13**A). Before removing the saw, a 2.2 (children and adolescents) or 2.5 (adults) K-wire is driven from distal through the calcaneocuboid joint and the calcaneal neck until it reaches the saw blade (see **Fig. 13**B). The osteotomy is now complete, and a Hintermann spreader is installed to open the osteotomy (see **Fig. 13**C). The spreader is opened until enough correction of the hindfoot valgus, the planus, and the forefoot abduction component is reached. Meanwhile, an iliac crest bone wedge is harvested, cut to the required size, and impacted into the opened osteotomy (see **Fig. 13**D). The 2.2 K-wire, inserted earlier, can now easily be driven forward into the posterior part of the calcaneus (see

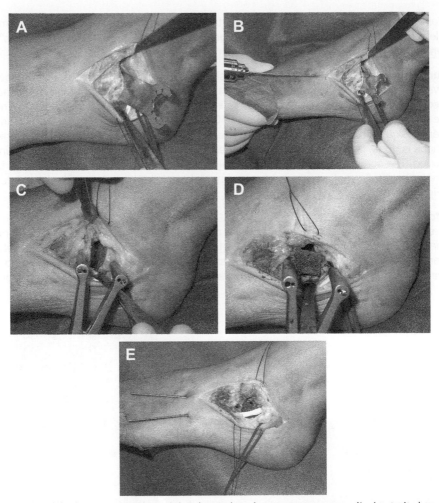

Fig. 13. Modified Evans procedure. (*A*) Calcaneal neck osteotomy perpendicular to its longitudinal axis at least 1 cm proximal to the calcaneocuboid joint. (*B*) A K-wire is drilled through the cuboid bone, the calcaneocuboid joint, and the distal part of the calcaneal neck until it reaches the saw blade. (*C*) After application of a Hintermann spreader, the osteotomy is opened till the needed correction is achieved. (*D*) An iliac crest bone wedge is impacted. (*E*) The osteotomy and the wedge are fixed with three to four crossing K-wires.

Fig. 13E). This step is followed by inserting two or three more K-wires (two from anterior, one to two from posterior) and performing a radiographic check. Alternatively, an angle-stable locking compression plate can be used in adults.

Calcaneocuboid distraction-fusion
This technique is an alternative to the Evans procedure and is considered in adults or in the case of instability or arthritis of the calcaneocuboid joint. In older patients who have neurogenic planovalgus foot in which lateral column lengthening is indicated, this technique is preferred over the Evans procedure.

The approach is done in a slightly S-shaped style over the calcaneocuboid joint, and the sural nerve is retracted. The extensor digitorum brevis is released from the anterior process of the calcaneus, and the calcaneocuboid joint is exposed (**Fig. 14A**). All the cartilage is removed with a chisel using the sparing technique (see **Fig. 14B**). Afterward, a Hintermann spreader is installed and opened (see **Fig. 14C, D**). The correction should then be checked clinically (see **Fig. 14E**). With the spreader, an exact correction can be chosen. The size of the wedge is measured. Transplantation of the wedge and the fixation of the fusion and the wedge are analogous to the Evans procedure, with crossing K-wires (see **Fig. 14F, G**) or an angle-stable locking plate.

Grice procedure
A slightly dorsally S-shaped skin incision is done over the sinus tarsi.[11] The sural nerve and the peroneal tendons are identified and retracted. The neck of the calcaneus is exposed, and the sinus tarsi is freed from fat (**Fig. 15A**). The foot is held in hindfoot eversion. A small flat chisel is inserted between the distal aspect of the calcaneal neck and the talus. The chisel is then rotated. This maneuver is repeated with a broader chisel until all soft tissue is removed from the surfaces (see **Fig. 15B**). The foot is then brought into the corrected position, and the size of the needed bone graft is determined. After harvesting the bone wedge, it is prepared to the required size and is inserted (see **Fig. 15C, D**). Afterward, the wedge is fixed with three to four crossing K-wires (two from posterior, two from anterior, **Fig. 15E**). Preoperative and 2-years' post-Grice procedure radiographs of a 7-year-old diplegic patient are shown in **Fig. 15F and G**, respectively.

Gleich procedure
An incision is done over the tuber calcanei.[2] In the case of a previous Grice, Evans, or calcaneocuboid distraction osteotomy, the skin incision is lengthened posteriorly (**Fig. 16A**). The tuber calcanei is then subperiostally exposed by the insertion of two Hohmann levers (see **Fig. 16B**). Afterward, the osteotomy is performed with an oscillating bone saw perpendicular to the longitudinal axis of the tuber calcanei (see **Fig. 16C**). Completion of the osteotomy is checked with a flat chisel, which is inserted into the osteotomy and tilted (see **Fig. 16D**). The posterior part of the calcaneus is then shifted medially and plantar (see **Fig. 16E**). In this position, transfixation is done with two 2.2 K-wires in children and adolescents. In adults, two parallel cannulated screws for fixation are considered.

Triple fusion
This procedure is indicated for severe planovalgus feet, especially in adults and in those who have neurogenic disorders.

Chopart's fusion is performed using the standard approach (see the section "Charcot-Marie-Tooth disease and cavovarus foot"). The posterior tibial tendon is tagged and released (**Fig. 17A**). It is readapted under tension at the end of the operation. The capsule of the talonavicular joint is incised, and the cartilage is removed (see

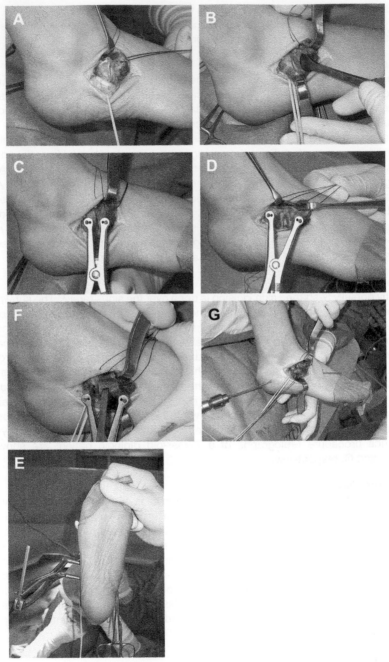

Fig. 14. Calcaneocuboid distraction-arthrodesis. (*A*) After release of the short extensor digitorum origin, the calcaneocuboid joint is exposed. (*B*) The cartilage is removed using the sparing convex–concave technique. (*C*) The Hintermann spreader is applied. (*D, E*) The joint can be opened until needed correction is achieved. (*F*) A prepared iliac crest bone wedge is impacted, which is followed by (*G*) transfixation with three to four crossing K-wires.

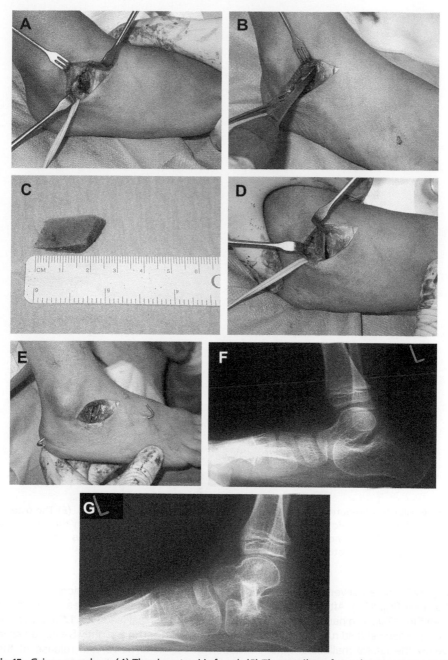

Fig. 15. Grice procedure. (*A*) The sinus tarsi is freed. (*B*) The cartilage from the anterior aspect of the subtalar joint is removed. (*C*) An adequate iliac crest bone wedge is prepared and (*D*) inserted between the calcaneus and talus. (*E*) Afterward, transfixation is done with two to four crossing K-wires. (*F*) Preoperative and (*G*) 2-year post Grice procedure lateral-view radiographs of a 7-year-old diplegic patient.

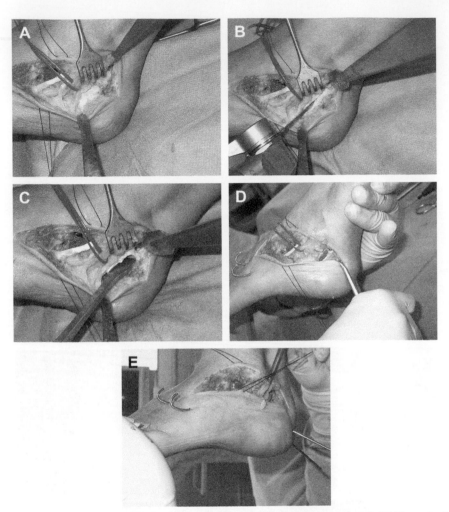

Fig. 16. Gleich procedure. (*A*) The tuber calcaneus is subperiostally exposed. (*B*) The osteotomy is done perpendicular to the longitudinal axis of the calcaneus with the oscillating bone saw. (*C*) It is opened with a chisel. (*D*) The dorsal part of the calcaneus is then shifted medially. (*E*) The osteotomy is fixed with two to three K-wires or screws.

Fig. 17B). In very severe cases, additional naviculectomy is needed to achieve correction (see **Fig. 17**C). After navicular bone resection, the cuneiform bones can be seen (see **Fig. 17**D). The cartilage is then removed with the chisel (see **Fig. 17**E). Laterally, the approach should run over the calcaneocuboid joint and in a slightly S-shaped style below the lateral malleolus. After retraction of the sural nerve and release of the extensor digitorum brevis muscle, the calcaneocuboid and subtalar joints are exposed by the insertion of Viernstein levers (see **Fig. 17**F, G). All ligaments in the subtalar space are dissected and all cartilage is removed from the calcaneocuboid and subtalar joints using the sparing technique (see **Fig. 17**H). The foot is then redressed into a corrected position and initially fixed at the talonavicular joint with two K-wires. Afterward, a spreader is inserted into the subtalar space and opened. The next step is the transfixation of the calcaneocuboid joint with two more K-wires. The amount of

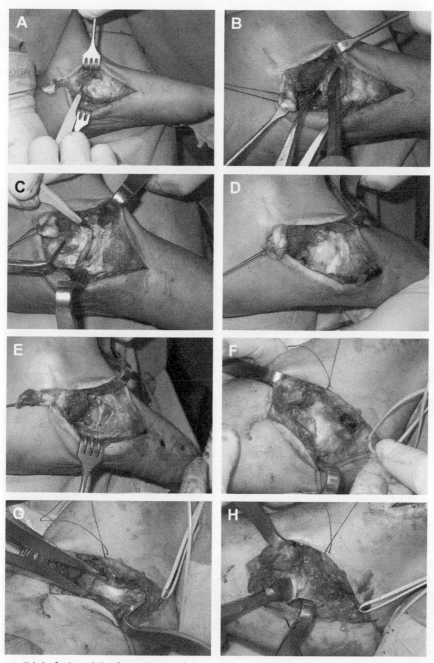

Fig. 17. Triple fusion. (*A*) After release of the posterior tibial tendon, the capsule of the talo-navicular joint is incised. (*B*) Cartilage is removed from the navicular bone and the talus head. (*C*) In some cases of severe planovalgus with an extremely short lateral border, navi-culectomy may be needed. (*D, E*) In such cases, the cuneiform bones are fused with the talus. All the cartilage is resected. (*F–H*) Lateral views showing that the calcaneocuboid joint and the subtalar joint are freed from cartilage.

a lateral-based wedge is determined and is harvested from the iliac crest. The spreader is removed, and the wedge is inserted into the subtalar space. Two additional K-wires are drilled in for the fixation of calcaneus, wedge, and talus. The wires can be inserted from plantar posterior in a parallel technique or in a crossing technique. In older patients or in those who have the previously named risk factors for nonunion, cannulated compression screws should be used.

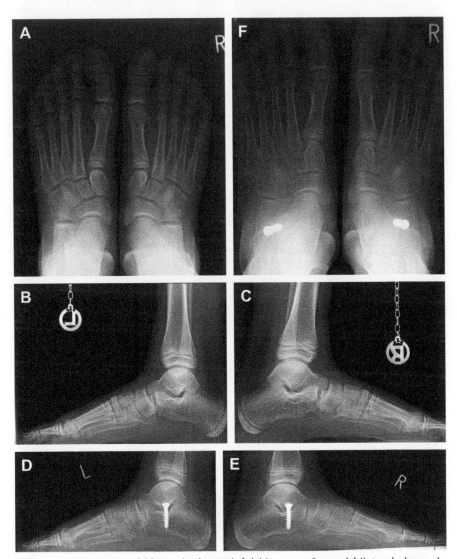

Fig. 18. Case 1: a 13-year-old boy who has painful (since age 2 years) bilateral planovalgus foot (nonneurologic) not improved by conservative treatment. Preoperative lateral-view (*A*) and AP-view (*B*, *C*) radiographs. Follow-up lateral-view (*D*, *E*) and AP-view (*F*) radiographs at 6 months. Patient has persistent pain in the right foot; left foot is asymptomatic. (*G*) Lateral-view radiograph at 5 weeks post combined Evans and Gleich procedure (*right side*). One-year follow-up lateral-view (*H*) and AP-view (*I*) radiographs. Patient has no further pain.

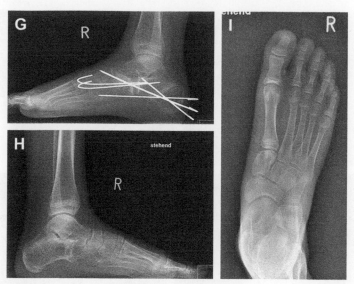

Fig. 18. (*continued*)

If necessary, calf muscle lengthening (Baumann,[28] Strayer,[29] and TAL), peroneal muscle lengthening, or flexor digitorum longus transfer to posterior tibial tendon[38] should be performed after the bony correction.

Postoperative Treatment

For postoperative treatment, see the section "Charcot-Marie-Tooth disease and cavovarus foot."

Outcome

Case 1
A 13-year-old boy presented with painful bilateral planovalgus foot (nonneurologic) (**Fig. 18**A–C). He suffered pain for over 2 years, which was not improved with conservative treatment. He underwent minimally invasive surgery with calcaneal–stop screw technique bilaterally. Four weeks after surgery, the boy was free from all pain. After 6 months, he returned and complained about persistent pain at the medial aspect of the right foot over the talonavicular joint from 1 month postoperatively. Radiographs showed an intact screw but a slightly increased valgus deformity on the right side (see **Fig. 18**D–F). Therefore, the screw was explanted, and an Evans and a Gleich osteotomy and calf muscle lengthening were performed in the same session (**Fig. 18**G shows results 5 weeks postoperatively). The patient is now free from all pain at 11 months since the second surgery (**Fig. 18**H, I).

Case 2
In the preoperative examination, a 15-year-old boy suffered from a severe planovalgus foot on the right side (**Fig. 19**A, B, in heel rise). He had pain over the navicular bone and the plantar fascia. The preoperative radiograph (see **Fig. 19**C) showed a severe planus component, subluxation of the talonavicular joint, and forefoot abduction. In the clinical examination, a severe instability of Chopart's joint was found. For this reason, the patient was treated with Chopart's fusion and an additive subtalar fusion (wedge implantation from lateral). Five-week postoperative radiographs are shown in

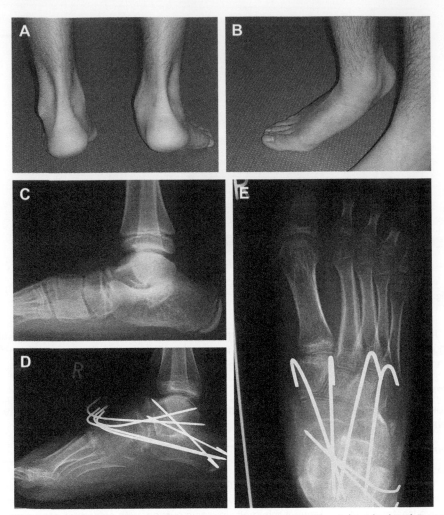

Fig.19. Case 2: a 15-year-old boy who has severe planovalgus on the right side. (*A, B*) Preoperative clinical manifestations in heel rise position. (*C*) Preoperative lateral-view radiograph. Lateral-view (*D*) and AP-view (*E*) radiographs at 5 weeks post surgery. (*F, G*) Two-year clinical follow-up. Lateral-view (*H*) and AP-view (*I*) follow-up radiographs at 2 years.

Fig. 19D, E. In this healthy young patient, K-wires were used for fixation (two talonavicular, two calcaneocuboid, and two talocalcaneal with wedge fixation). The patient is now free of any pain. He returned for a 2-year follow-up; the clinical and radiologic outcome is shown in **Fig. 19**F–I.

Case 3
Fig. 20 shows pre- and postoperative radiograhs of a 42-year-old woman who had a severe and painful planovalgus foot (AAFD) on the right side. A talonavicular fusion with calcaneocuboid lengthening fusion was performed and led to a nice correction of the hindfoot. Intraoperatively, a hyperextended first ray was seen and a flexion osteotomy of the first metatarsal was performed. Due to a positive smoker anamnesis, three angle-stable locking plates (Darco) were used for the fixation. The 1-year follow-up

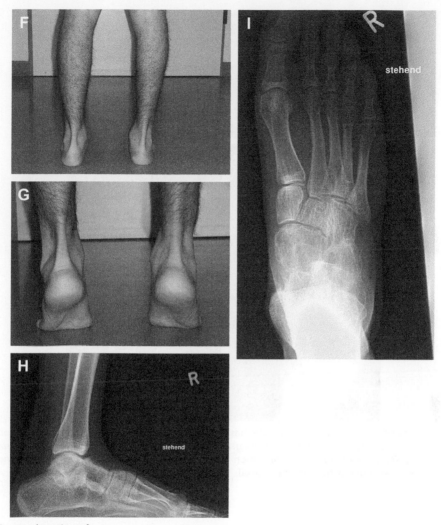

Fig. 19. (*continued*)

radiographs are shown in **Fig. 20**C, D. The patient is free of pain and able to wear regular shoes again.

Case 4

This case of a 54-year-old man who had AAFD due to an unknown neuropathic disorder and a positive history for nonunion (**Fig. 21**A) shows that K-wire fixation can be combined with angle-stable locking plates for additional stability. A triple fusion with subtalar wedge implantation and a first tarsometatarsal joint fusion were performed (**Fig. 21**B, 6 weeks postoperatively). The primary stabilization was done by way of K-wires. For compression in the talonavicular joint and the first tarsometatarsal joint, Charlotte™ Claw® compression plates (Wright Medical Technology, Inc., Arlington, VA) were used. After implantation, the middle part of these plates can be distracted, which compresses the osteotomy or fusion.

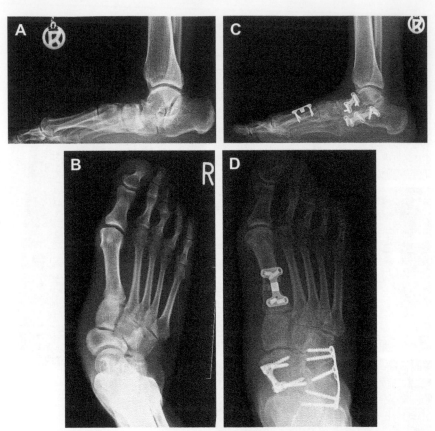

Fig. 20. Case 3: a 42-year-old woman who has severe and painful planovalgus foot (AAFD) on the right side. Lateral- and AP-view radiographs taken preoperatively (*A, B*) and at 1-year follow-up (*C, D*) after talonavicular fusion with calcaneocuboid lengthening fusion and a flexion osteotomy of the first metatarsal.

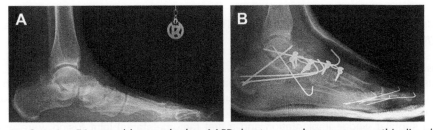

Fig. 21. Case 4: a 54-year-old man who has AAFD due to an unknown neuropathic disorder and a positive history for nonunion. Preoperative (*A*) and 6-week postoperative (*B*) lateral-view radiographs. The primary stabilization was done with Kirschner wires. For compression in the talonavicular joint and the first TMT joint, Charlotte Claw plates (Wright Medical) were used. After implantation, the middle part of these plates can be distracted, which compresses the osteotomy or fusion.

RECONSTRUCTION OF CHARCOT'S FOOT
Charcot's Foot: Etiology and Pathomechanics

Diabetes is the most common cause of Charcot's foot syndrome. Statistics from the American Diabetes Association show that 7% of the United States population (~21 million people) suffer from diabetes.[48] Every year, about 80,000 amputations have to be performed in diabetic patients. Patients who have diabetes have a 10 times higher risk for amputation than the nondiabetic population.

Neuropathy is one of the most common concomitant comorbidities of diabetes.[49] About 75% of patients who have diabetes suffer from neuropathy, which usually appears first in the distal part of the lower extremities.[50] In diabetic neuropathy, there is commonly a combination of motoric, sensory, and autonomic deficits.[51] The neuropathy causes weakness of the intrinsic foot muscles and can lead to contractures. Above all, the Achilles tendon can be affected, leading to contracture and equinus.[52] In equinus deformity, the pressure on the fore- and midfoot is increased. Positive results following TAL on recurrent ulceration and healing have been reported.[53]

All these factors in combination with vascular deficits lead to the typical Charcot's foot deformity (also called Charcot's joint, neuropathic osteoarthropathy), which is characterized by bony destruction, bone resorption, and various deformities. The first report of a diabetic patient who also had Charcot's foot appeared in 1936.[54] The incidence of Charcot's foot in diabetic patients ranges from 1% to 37%.[55,56]

Charcot's Foot: Classifications

Eichenholtz[57] was the first to report a staging method for Charcot's foot. He described three stages: acute, subacute (coalescence), and chronic (consolidation). The anatomic classification of Charcot's foot describes three types (**Table 7**).[58] **Fig. 22**A) illustrates a radiograph of a type I Charcot's foot. A typical radiograph of a 68-year-old man who has Charcot's, hindfoot equinus deformity, and consecutive midfoot break (type II and IIIA) is shown in **Fig. 22**B.

Charcot's Foot: Salvage Reconstructions of the Mid- and Hindfoot

Surgical reconstructive methods are limited to type III Charcot's foot. The principles of reconstruction are

Careful preoperative decision making
Extensive preoperative vascular, neurologic, and internal medicine examinations

Table 7			
Anatomic classification of Charcot's foot			
Type	Incidence	Localization	Problems
I	60%	Midfoot, tarsometatarsal, naviculocuneiform	Arch collapse, plantar medial exostosis, ulceration
II	30%–35%	Hindfoot	Instability, deformity, foot subluxation, ulceration
IIIA	5%	Ankle	Instability, deformity, ulceration
IIIB	5%	Fracture of calcaneal tuberosity	Weak push-off, planovalgus, ulceration

Data from Brodsky JW, Kwong PK, Wagner FW, et al. Patterns of breakdown in the Charcot tarsus of diabetes and relation to treatment. Orthop Trans 1987;2:484.

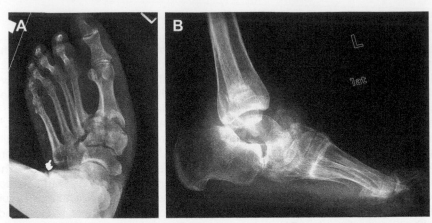

Fig. 22. Typical manifestations of Charcot's arthropathy. The anatomic classification of Charcot's foot describes three types (see Table 7). (*A*) AP-view radiograph of type I Charcot's foot. (*B*) Typical radiograph of a type II+IIIA Charcot's foot (hindfoot equinus deformity and consecutive midfoot break).

Removal of all low-quality bone and disturbing soft tissue

Reconstruction of the bony structure with iliac crest bone wedges (or other autologous material)

Solid osteosynthesis using long angle-stable locking plates, screws, nails, or external fixation systems

Cautious skin closure; plastic surgical reconstruction if necessary

Surgical Technique

Case 1 (ankle fusion, angle-stable locking plates)

Fig. 23A–D shows the preoperative clinical and radiographic state of a 58-year-old woman who has diabetes mellitus type 2 and rheumatoid arthritis. Over the last 2 years she nearly lost her walking ability due to increasing instability and deformity of her right foot. The preoperative pictures show an extreme planovalgus deformity with kissing medial malleolus sign (the medial malleolus kisses the ground) and severe instability (see **Fig. 23**A, B). A totally destroyed midfoot and hindfoot was evident on the radiographs (see **Fig. 23**C, D). The distal tibia has driven the talus through the anterior calcaneus and the midfoot to the sole of the foot. The instability in the ankle and subtalar joint has led to severe valgus. Due to the age of the patient, the working blood supply, and the relatively good skin condition, salvage reconstructive surgery was a promising alternative to amputation. The patient underwent reconstructive surgery with resection of the fibula, talus, anterior calcaneus, midfoot, and all tendons (see **Fig. 23**E). A combined lateral and medial approach was chosen. Afterward, the distal tibia was resected with the oscillating bone saw (see **Fig. 23**F). The cranial parts of the calcaneus were also resected until vital bone occurred. Large iliac crest bone wedges were taken and inserted between the forefoot and the calcaneus. They were temporarily fixed with K-wires. Then, the distal tibia was fitted to the surface of the calcaneus and also temporarily fixed. Afterward, two distal tibial angle-stable locking plates (less invasive stabilization system) were installed, one from lateral, the other from anterior (see **Fig. 23**G). The patient was treated with a non-weight-bearing cast for 8 weeks. After this time, a weight-bearing cast was put on, starting with 20% of body load. The load was increased over time and after 12 weeks, 100% was reached. After 12

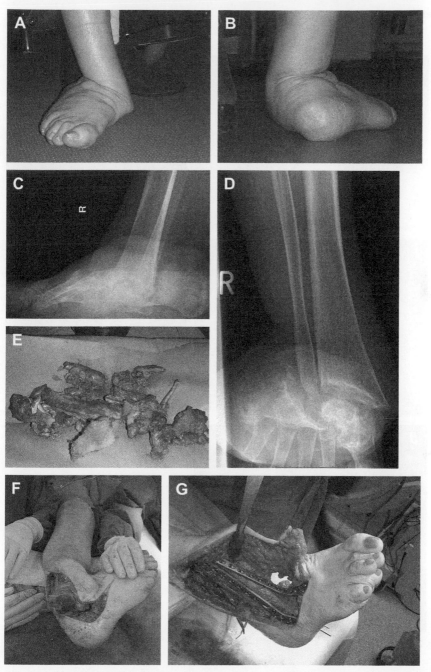

Fig. 23. Case 1: a 58-year-old woman who has diabetes mellitus type 2 and rheumatoid arthritis. (*A, B*) Preoperative clinical manifestations: extreme planovalgus deformity with kissing medial malleolus sign (the medial malleolus kisses the ground) and severe instability. Preoperative lateral-view (*C*) and AP-view (*D*) radiographs. (*E*) The patient underwent reconstructive surgery with resection of the fibula, talus, anterior calcaneus, midfoot, and all tendons. (*F*) The distal tibia was resected with the oscillating bone saw. (*G*) Two distal tibial angle-stable locking plates (less invasive stabilization system) were installed, one from lateral, the other from anterior, fusing the distal tibia with the remaining calcaneus, the large bone wedges, and the cuneiform bones. (*H, I*) Ten-month clinical follow-up. Ten-month follow-up lateral-view (*J*) and AP-view (*K*) radiographs.

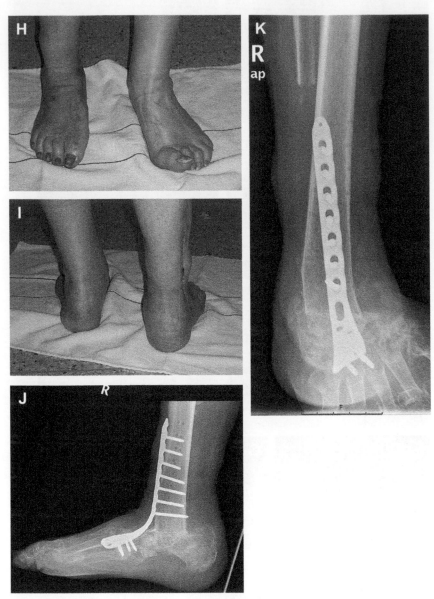

Fig. 23. (*continued*)

weeks, the patient walked in an orthopedic shoe. Meanwhile, the lateral plate had to be removed because of skin problems. After hardware removal, the wound healed. Ten months after surgery, the patient returned for follow-up (see **Fig. 23**H–K).

Case 2 (cannulated screws)

Fig. 24 shows the preoperative and 10-month postoperative radiographs of a 68-year-old man who has diabetes and type II Charcot's foot. The patient suffered from a severe planovalgus foot and ulceration at the medial border of the foot. A triple fusion with partial resection of the talus and the navicular bone was performed. Iliac crest wedges were harvested and fitted to the defect in Chopart's line. The triple fusion was fixed with six cannulated screws (see **Fig. 24**C, D). The ulceration healed completely.

Case 3 (angle-stable locking plates midfoot)

Fig. 25 shows the preoperative and 1-year postoperative radiographs of a 45-year-old man who has diabetes and type I Charcot's foot. The patient had ulceration several years at the medial border of the foot. He was offered an amputation in another hospital. Furthermore, he was disabled by the limited walking distance due to severe pain in the midfoot. Salvage surgery with resection of the whole midfoot was performed (see **Fig. 25**B). Big bone wedges were harvested from both iliac crests, implanted into the midfoot and temporarily fixed with K-wires. After reconstruction of the bony structure of the midfoot, three angle-stable locking plates were used to fix the whole midfoot to the hindfoot and forefoot. Approximately 1 year after surgery, the bone has healed (see **Fig. 25**C) and the patient is able to walk long distances with orthopedic shoes and without pain.

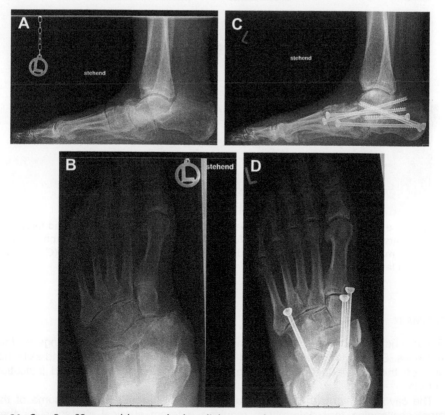

Fig. 24. Case 2: a 68-year-old man who has diabetes and type II Charcot's foot (severe plano-valgus foot and ulceration at the medial border of the foot). Preoperative lateral-view (*A*) and AP-view (*B*) radiographs. Ten-month follow-up lateral-view (*C*) and AP-view (*D*) radiographs.

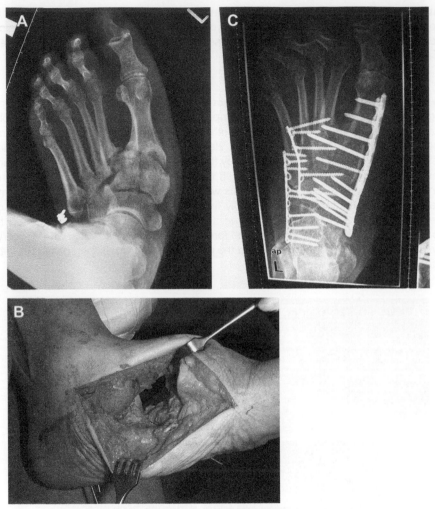

Fig. 25. Case 3: a 45-year-old man who has diabetes, type I Charcot's foot, and ulceration several years at the medial border of the foot. (*A*) Preoperative lateral radiograph. (*B*) Intraoperative massive bony defect after wide resection of poor quality bone. (*C*) One-year follow-up lateral-view radiograph.

SUMMARY

Reconstruction surgery of the mid- and hindfoot is a demanding challenge for foot surgeons. Satisfactory results depend not only on surgical technique and skills but also on the knowledge of underlying disorders, pathomechanics, and indication criteria.

The cavovarus foot, the planovalgus foot, and Charcot's foot are some of the most challenging foot deformities, requiring different surgical strategies for their correction. Most of the osteotomies and fusions in children and adults can be fixed with transcutaneous K-wires, which are inexpensive, easy to use, and remove easily without general anesthesia after 4 weeks (children) or 6 weeks (adults), depending on bone healing. Special indications, depending on age, vascular situation, risk for nonunion, and underlying pathology (eg, Charcot's foot), demand alternative fixation systems such as cannulated screws, compression screws, or angle-stable locking plates.

REFERENCES

1. Wenz W, Dreher T. Charcot-Marie-Tooth disease and the cavovarus foot. In: Pinzur MS, editor. Orthopaedic knowledge update—foot and ankle. Rosemont, IL: AAOS; 2008. p. 291–306.
2. Gleich A. Beitrag zur operativen Plattfußbehandlung [Contribution to the treatment of planovalgus]. Arch Klin Chir 1893;46:358–62 [in German].
3. Koutsogiannis E. Treatment of mobile flat foot by displacement osteotomy of the calcaneus. J Bone Joint Surg Br 1971;53:96–100.
4. Evans D. Calcaneo-valgus deformity. J Bone Joint Surg Br 1987;57:270–8.
5. Zwipp H, Rammelt S. Modified Evans osteotomy for the operative treatment of acquired pes planovalgus. Oper Orthop Traumatol 2006;2:182–97.
6. Cole WH. The treatment of claw-foot. J Bone Joint Surg 1940;22:895–908.
7. McHale KA, Lenhart MK. Treatment of residual clubfoot deformity—the "bean shaped" foot—by opening wedge medial cuneiform osteotomy and closing wedge cuboid osteotomy. Clinical review and cadaver correlations. J Pediatr Orthop 1991;11:374–81.
8. Toksvig-Larsen S, Ryd L, Lindstrand A. On the problem of heat generation in bone cutting. Studies on the effects on liquid cooling. J Bone Joint Surg Br 1991;73:13–5.
9. Lambrinudi C. New operation on drop foot. Br J Surg 1927;15:193–200.
10. Wenz W, Bruckner T, Akbar M. Complete tendon transfer and inverse Lambrinudi arthrodesis: preliminary results of a new technique for the treatment of paralytic pes calcaneus. Foot Ankle Int 2008;29:683–9.
11. Grice DS. An extra-articular arthrodesis of the sub-astragalar joint for the correction of paralytic flat feet in children. J Bone Joint Surg Am 1952;34:927–40.
12. Skre H. Genetic and clinical aspects of Charcot-Marie-Tooth's disease. Clin Genet 1974;6:98–118.
13. Lupski JR, de Oca-Luna RM, Slaugenhaupt S, et al. DNA duplication associated with Charcot-Marie-Tooth disease type 1A. Cell 1991;66:219.
14. Wines AP, Chen D, Lynch B, et al. Foot deformities in children with hereditary motor and sensory neuropathy. J Pediatr Orthop 2005;25:241–4.
15. Nagai MK, Chan G, Guille JT, et al. Prevalence of Charcot-Marie-Tooth disease in patients who have bilateral cavovarus feet. J Pediatr Orthop 2006;26:438–43.
16. Berger P, Niemann A, Suter U. Schwann cells and the pathogenesis of inherited motor and sensory neuropathies (Charcot-Marie-Tooth disease). Glia 2006;54:243–57.
17. Berger P, Young P, Suter U. Molecular cell biology of Charcot-Marie-Tooth disease. Neurogenetics 2002;4:1–15.
18. Holmes JR, Hansen ST. Foot and ankle manifestations of Charcot Marie Tooth disease. Foot Ankle 1993;14:476–86.
19. Mann RA, Missirian J. Pathophysiology of Charcot-Marie-Tooth disease. Clin Orthop Relat Res 1988;234:221–8.
20. Brady RO, Schiffmann R. Clinical features of and recent advances in therapy for Fabry disease. JAMA 2000;284:2771–5.
21. Pareyson D. Diagnosis of hereditary neuropathies in adult patients. J Neurol 2003;250:148–60.

22. Metaxiotis D, Accles W, Pappas A, et al. Dynamic pedobarography (DPB) in operative management of cavovarus foot deformity. Foot Ankle Int 2000;21: 935–47.

23. Simon J, Doederlein L, McIntosh AS, et al. The Heidelberg foot measurement method: development, description and assessment. Gait Posture 2006;23: 411–24.

24. Steindler A. The treatment of pes cavus (hollow claw foot). Arch Surg 1921;2: 325–37.

25. Tubby AH. Deformities including diseases of bones and joints. 2nd edition. London: MacMillan; 1912.

26. Hsu JD, Hoffer MM. Posterior tibial tendon transfer anteriorly through the interosseus membrane. Clin Orthop 1978;131:202–4.

27. Dwyer FC. The present status of the problem of pes cavus. Clin Orthop 1975;106: 254–75.

28. Baumann JU, Koch HG. Ventrale aponeurotische Verlängerung des Musculus gastrocnemius [Anterior aponeurotic lengthening of gastrocnemius muscle]. Oper Orthop Traumatol 1989;4:254–8.

29. Strayer LM. Gastrocnemius recession: a five-year report of cases. J Bone Joint Surg Am 1958;40:1019–30 [in German].

30. Jones R. An operation for paralytic calcaneo-cavus. Am J Orthop Surg 1908;5: 371–6.

31. DePalma L, Colonna E, Travasi M. The modified Jones procedure for pes cavovarus with claw hallux. J Foot Ankle Surg 1997;36:279–83.

32. Vlachou M, Beris A, Dimitriadis D. Modified Chuinard-Baskin procedure for managing mild-to-moderate cavus and claw foot deformity in children and adolescents. J Foot Ankle Surg 2008;47(4):313–20.

33. Barbari SG, Brevig K. Correction of clawtoes by the Girdlestone-Taylor flexor-extensor transfer procedure. Foot Ankle 1984;5(2):67–73.

34. Chan G, Sampath J, Miller F, et al. The role of the dynamic pedobarography in assessing treatment of cavovarus feet in children with Charcot-Marie-Tooth disease. J Pediatr Orthop 2007;27:510–6.

35. Azmaipairashvili Z, Riddle EC, Scavina M, et al. Correction of cavovarus foot deformity in Charcot-Marie-Tooth disease. J Pediatr Orthop 2005;25:360–5.

36. Wetmore RS, Drennan JC. Long-term results of triple arthrodesis in Charcot-Marie-Tooth disease. J Bone Joint Surg Am 1989;71:417–22.

37. Roth S, Sestan B, Tudor A, et al. Minimally invasive calcaneal-stop method for idiopathic flexible pes planovalgus in children. Foot Ankle Int 2007;28:991–5.

38. Marks RM, Long JT, Ness ME, et al. Surgical reconstruction of posterior tibial tendon dysfunction: prospective comparison of flexor digitorum longus substitution combined with lateral column lengthening or medial displacement calcaneal osteotomy. Gait Posture 2009;29:17–22.

39. Jones A. An operation for paralytic calcaneo-cavus. Am J Orthop Surg 1908;5: 371–6.

40. Staheli L, Chew D, Corbett M. The longitudinal arch. A survey of eight hundred and eighty-two feet in normal children and adults. J Bone Joint Surg 1987;69A:426–8.

41. Harris RI, Beath T. Hypermobile flat-foot with short tendo achilles. J Bone Joint Surg 1948;30:116–38.

42. Mann R, Inman VT. Phasic activity of intrinsic muscles of the foot. J Bone Joint Surg Am 1964;46:469–81.

43. Basmajian JV, Stecko G. The role of muscles in arch supports of the foot. J Bone Joint Surg Am 1963;45:1184–90.

44. Jack EA. Naviculo-cuneiform fusion in the treatment of flat foot. J Bone Joint Surg Br 1953;35:75–82.
45. Myerson MS. Adult acquired flatfoot deformity. J Bone Joint Surg 1996;78: 780–90.
46. Needleman RL. A surgical approach for flexible flatfeet in adults including a sub-talar arthroereisis with the MBA sinus tarsi implant. Foot Ankle Int 2006;27(1): 9–18.
47. Scher DM, Bansal M, Handler-Matasar S, et al. Extensive implant reaction in failed subtalar joint arthroereisis: report of two cases. HSS J 2007;3(2):177–81.
48. American Diabetes Association. Diabetes—statistics. Available at: http://www.diabetes.org/diabetes-statistics.jsp; 2007. Accessed June 11, 2009.
49. Adler A. Risk factors for diabetic neuropathy and foot ulceration. Curr Diab Rep 2001;1:202–7.
50. Ross MA. Neuropathies associated with diabetes. Med Clin North Am 1993;77: 111–24.
51. Ischii DN. Implications of insulin-like growth factors in the pathogenesis of dia-betic neuropathy. Brain Res Rev 1995;20:47–67.
52. Lin SS, Lee TH, Wapner KL. Plantar forefoot ulceration with equinus deformity of the ankle in diabetic patients: the effect of tendo-Achilles lengthening and total contact casting. Orthopaedics 1996;19:465–75.
53. Mueller MJ, Sinacore DR, Hastings MK, et al. Effect of Achilles tendon length-ening on neuropathic plantar ulcers: a randomized clinical trial. J Bone Joint Surg Am 2003;85:1436–45.
54. Jordan W. Neuritic manifestations in diabetes mellitus. Arch Intern Med 1936;57: 307–66.
55. Cavanagh PR, Young MJ, Adams JE, et al. Radiographic abnormalities in the feet of patients with diabetic neuropathies. Diabetes Care 1994;17:201–9.
56. Brodsky JW, Kwong PK, Wagner FW, et al. Patterns of breakdown in the Char-cot tarsus of diabetes and relation to treatment [abstract]. Orthop Trans 1987; 2:484.
57. Eichenholtz S. Charcot joints. Springfield (IL): Charles C. Thomas; 1966.
58. Bordsky JW. The diabetic foot. In: Coughlin MJ, Mann RA, Saltzmann CL, editors. Surgery of the foot and ankle. 8th edition. Philadelphia: Mosby; 2007. p. 1281–368.
59. Selber P, Filho ER, Dallalana R, et al. Supramalleolar derotation osteotomy of the tibia, with T plate fixation. Technique and results in patients with neuromus-cular disease. J Bone Joint Surg Br 2004;86:1170–5.
60. McNicol D, Leong JC, Hsu LC. Supramalleolar derotation osteotomy for lateral tibial torsion and associated equinovarus deformity of the foot. J Bone Joint Surg Br 1983;65:166–70.

Reconstruction of Multiplanar Ankle and Hindfoot Deformity with Intramedullary Techniques

George E. Quill, Jr., MD[a,b],*

KEYWORDS

- Multiplanar deformity • Hindfoot • Ankle
- Intramedullary fixation • Arthrodesis

Disabling ankle and hindfoot deformity presents in myriad forms and may be associated with various neuromuscular deficits and functional limitations that can be painful.[1–3] Multiplanar ankle and hindfoot deformity may result from primary osteoarthritis or rheumatoid arthritis and the sequelae of significant open or closed trauma.[4,5] Skeletal defects after tumor resection, failed prior reconstructive arthrodesis or arthroplasty techniques, and the sequelae of poliomyelitis, paraplegia, and hereditary sensorimotor deficits can provide challenges to the treating orthopaedic surgeon.[6–8] The goal of treatment always should to be to address the presenting concerns of the patient and the deformity and achieve a stable, functional, and hopefully pain-free plantigrade foot. These goals are accomplished by appropriate preoperative assessment of the patient and radiographic studies and meticulous preoperative planning with detailed attention to intraoperative surgical technique. Diligent aftercare and aggressive management of complications ensure the most optimal postoperative outcome.

PATIENT INTERVIEW

One of the most telling and helpful questions a surgeon may ask a patient is "If you could point with one finger to the area that bothers you the worst, what would you show me?" Localized pain is often mechanical or arthritic in etiology and is the type we can address most successfully. Generalized pain, neuritic pain, vascular

[a] Department of Orthopedic Surgery, University of Louisville School of Medicine, 530 S Jackson Street, Louisville, KY 40202, USA
[b] Louisville Orthopaedic Clinic, 4130 Dutchmans Lane, Louisville, KY 40207, USA
* Corresponding author.
E-mail address: Gboneq1@yahoo.com

Foot Ankle Clin N Am 14 (2009) 533–547
doi:10.1016/j.fcl.2009.05.001
1083-7515/09/$ – see front matter © 2009 Elsevier Inc. All rights reserved.

foot.theclinics.com

insufficiency, or neuropathic pain is difficult to improve with an operation. A good history is imperative in setting us on the path to the correct treatment and often elucidates whether the problem is caused by antecedent trauma or open or closed injury or whether primary arthritis is a concern. It is important to ascertain whether the patient's pain is present at rest or is activity related, whether there is radiation distally or proximally to this discomfort, and how it may impart upon gait pattern or the ipsilateral knee, hip, or back. When pain is worse on uneven ground than on level surfaces, the origin of the pain is often the subtalar joint or—slightly less commonly—the transverse tarsal joints.[9] The history of giving way is often present in a patient with an unstable ankle or fixed hindfoot varus, which also may be associated with peroneal insufficiency and weakness of eversion power (**Fig. 1**). A history of locking usually indicates the presence of an intra-articular loose body.

Shoewear limitations may be present, and one should ascertain whether the patient perceives an abnormal shoewear pattern. Determining the prior use and benefit, if any, from bracing, injections, and oral medications helps guide future treatment. Patients also may have proximal deformity that requires reconstruction. To ensure that the foot is positioned properly in space and in a plantigrade posture relative to the floor, any proximal realignment osteotomy or total knee arthroplasty should be performed before any ankle or hindfoot reconstruction.

Secondary to the potentially long postoperative recovery, it is important to ascertain whether a patient has help at home and whether the physical layout of the home is conducive to postoperative mobility. Consider the use of a scooter or wheelchair if a patient does not have the upper extremity strength to use crutches or a walker. Preoperative assessment with a physical therapist objectively determines the patient's ability to use an assistive device.

PATIENT EXAMINATION

A thorough musculoskeletal, neurologic, and vascular examination of the patient is critical. The surgeon must evaluate both lower extremities, the gait pattern, and the biomechanical axis of the involved limb. In addition to a careful musculoskeletal and neurologic examination, one should assess the location of calluses, ulcerations, scars, and soft tissue defects. Assessment of the wear pattern of the patient's current footwear can help determine subtle malalignment of the hindfoot. As an example, a patient

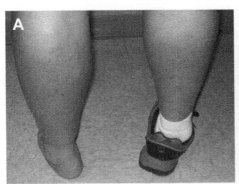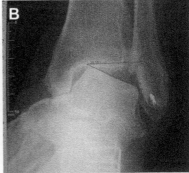

Fig. 1. Weight-bearing clinical photograph (*A*) and weight-bearing anteroposterior radiograph (*B*) of a 53-year-old laborer with persistent ankle and hindfoot varus instability after prior attempt at calcaneal osteotomy and lateral ligament reconstruction.

with a tendency to genu recurvatum in stance secondary to an equinus contracture or anterior tibiotalar abutment with discrete calluses on the plantar forefoot would most likely be comfortable in a higher heeled shoe to minimize the stress on the knee and place the ankle in the patient's functional range of motion (**Fig. 2**).

A patient with Charcot-Marie-Tooth disease typically has a varus hindfoot, peroneal muscle insufficiency, and a plantar-flexed first ray with a callus under the first metatarsal head.[1,10,11] The patient with severe hindfoot valgus has subfibular impingement, deltoid and posterior tibial tendon insufficiency, and fixed forefoot varus that must be taken into account when using intramedullary fixation for reconstruction.[3,12] If the forefoot deformities are passively correctable, then it may be possible to achieve a plantigrade foot without performing forefoot osteotomies or extending a hindfoot fusion mass to the midfoot in the form of an extended pantalar arthrodesis.[5]

PREOPERATIVE ASSESSMENT, INCLUDING RADIOGRAPHS AND ADDITIONAL DIAGNOSTIC TESTING

At a minimum, weight-bearing anteroposterior radiographs of the ankle and anteroposterior and lateral radiographs of the involved foot while standing should be obtained. These films should include as much of the distal tibia as necessary to visualize any existing hardware, malunited fractures, or other potential stress risers that may be present (**Fig. 3**). Additional special views, such as oblique or Harris-Beath views of the foot to assess for tarsal coalition, may be necessary. It is often helpful to obtain comparison radiographs of the contralateral uninvolved limb for preoperative

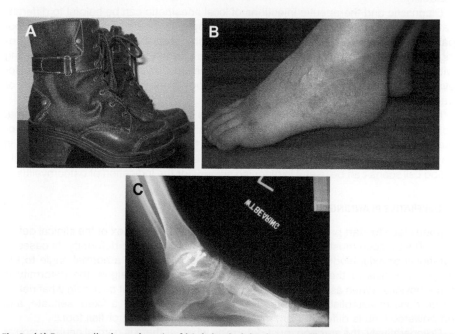

Fig. 2. (A) Reportedly the only pair of high-heeled, high-topped boots in which a 42-year-old woman was comfortable 2 years after sustaining bilateral talus fractures malunited in equinus. (B) Clinical appearance of the woman's foot in maximal passive left ankle dorsiflexion. (C) Weight-bearing lateral radiograph of the woman's foot. Note plantarflexion talus fracture malunion and posttraumatic osteoarthritis after open reduction and internal fixation.

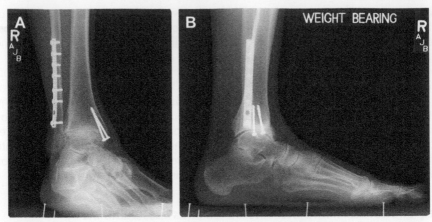

Fig. 3. Radiographs of the weight-bearing anteroposterior ankle (*A*) and lateral foot (*B*) of a 36-year-old man with posttraumatic osteoarthritis of the ankle.

purposes.[9] Often we radiograph the knee joint above the hindfoot to be reconstructed to assess for coronal plane abnormalities. We have found it helpful to get tangential views of the sesamoid on special occasions when assessing potential causes of forefoot discomfort because the sesamoids may be arthritic, fractured, or unduly proud if subluxed. Stress radiographs are helpful in elucidating ankle or syndesmotic instability.

Diagnostic and therapeutic injections of local anesthetic can be helpful to differentiate the anatomic source of pain.[12,13] For example, in a patient with lateral hindfoot pain, an injection in the sinus tarsi can distinguish between pains arising from pathologic peroneal tendons and pains attributable to an arthritic subtalar joint. CT scanning with both feet and ankles in the gantry at the same time is a useful preoperative tool for evaluating cases with suspected subtalar pathology, bone loss, neoplasia infection, or trauma (**Fig. 4**).

MRI helps greatly in ascertaining the presence or absence of bone marrow edema, soft tissue pathology, synovial proliferation, and tibiotalar avascular necrosis. Technetium nuclear medicine bone scans are sensitive tests that produce positive results in any situation that increases circulation to bone. Technetium- and indium-labeled white blood cell scans can be useful in planning surgery for the indication of osteomyelitis.[14]

PREOPERATIVE PLANNING

A good place to start preoperative planning is assessing the apex of the clinical deformity. The surgeon must assess the direction of the apex of the deformity. In cases of rotational or axial hindfoot malalignment, the foot may be at a normal angle to the longitudinal axis of the limb. In cases of severe varus or valgus, the deformity is more obvious. When assessing the deformity, the surgeon must ascertain what needs to be done to establish a plantigrade foot. The treatment for a fixed, sensate, and empowered limb is different from that for a flexible, insensate, or flail foot.

Preoperatively, the surgeon must determine whether there is normal neuromuscular function about the foot and ankle. Are the posterior tibial tendon and peroneal muscles and tendons functioning? Does the patient have a drop foot, persistence of a congenital or developmental deformity, or even a hereditary sensorimotor neuropathy or the sequelae of poliomyelitis? Another important clinical question is whether the subtalar

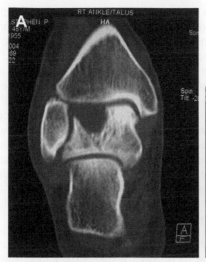
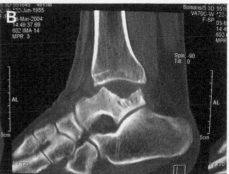

Fig. 4. Coronal (A) and lateral (B) CT images of a 48-year-old man with massive osteochondral talar insufficiency.

joint can be spared, especially when the surgeon is contemplating the use of intramedullary fixation for hindfoot reconstruction. Preoperatively, the surgeon must ensure that he or she has the appropriate instrumentation and personnel and intraoperative fluoroscopic imaging. The anesthetic technique should be considered carefully, as should positioning of the patient on the operating room table.

Finally, the surgeon should consider adjuvants for healing, including a bone graft that may be autograft, allograft, or synthetic. One may consider either external or implanted electrical bone stimulation to improve healing rates. Currently, one also must strongly consider using available orthobiologic adjuvants for optimal healing. The surgeon may choose from platelet-derived autologous growth factors, bone marrow aspirate, demineralized bone matrix, and even bone morphogenetic protein. All of the factors mentioned in this section are carefully considered preoperatively and impact the operative technique to be discussed in the next section. Specifically, the surgeon must consider preoperatively the advantages, disadvantages, indications, and contraindications of intramedullary fixation techniques in reconstructing ankle and hindfoot deformity.

The advantages of medullary nail fixation for ankle and hindfoot reconstruction include the fact that intramedullary nails are load-sharing devices that are especially useful in the treatment of osteopenic patients and they provide excellent early stability, ensuring position and alignment from the beginning.[5,15] Medullary nail fixation devices are also advantageous compared to more traditional methods of fixation because often a shorter period of postoperative immobilization and activity restriction is required.[7,11,16] Intramedullary fixation is advantageous for neuroarthropathic patients or patients who have insufficiency of the distal tibia, talus, or calcaneus.[6,17]

Medullary nail fixation is indicated for cases of arthrodesis in which there has been avascular necrosis of the talus, failed ankle replacement with subtalar intrusion, or a failed ankle fusion with insufficient talar body.[6,18–24] Other indications include primary or secondary osteoarthrosis, rheumatoid arthritis, the sequelae of trauma (especially distal tibial pilon fractures), and management of patients with neuromuscular disease, pseudarthrosis, neuroarthropathy, or skeletal defects after tumor resection.[1–7,10–13,15,17,25–33]

Medullary nail contraindications include the dysvascular extremity or one in which there is a severe active infection.[14] Relative contraindications to medullary nail fixation include insufficient plantar padding because most of the devices are inserted in retrograde fashion through the heel. The surgeon should think twice about passing a medullary nail across an otherwise normal subtalar joint except in cases in which it is worthwhile to fuse the subtalar joint and the ankle during the same operative procedure because of avascular necrosis of the talus, talar insufficiency, or distal tibial insufficiency caused by prior trauma or tumor resection. In these cases it would be acceptable to fuse an otherwise normal subtalar joint in order to span the diseased more proximal bone with an intramedullary fixation device. Even severe, fixed angular deformities of the distal tibia, ankle, and hindfoot can be overcome with periarticular osteotomies that make a collinear reduction of the tibia, ankle, and hindfoot possible in order to pass a retrograde intramedullary nail.[5,12]

INTRAOPERATIVE TECHNIQUE: AUTHOR'S PREFERRED METHODS

The general principles of intramedullary fixation for hindfoot and ankle reconstruction are as follows. The surgeon's goal should be to achieve a plantigrade foot while relieving pain, correcting deformity, and producing a solid fusion. A plantigrade foot is defined as one that is held at approximately 90° to the long axis of the tibia and in no more than 5° to 7° of hindfoot valgus. In stance, a plantigrade foot is one in which a tripod of weight bearing, including the heel and the first and fifth metatarsal heads, is achieved simultaneously.[34–36] The first and fifth metatarsal heads must strike the ground together in stance. Equinus leads to genu recurvatum and early heel off. Patients with an equinus malunion walk with external rotation of the hip (**Fig. 5**). Dorsiflexion is better tolerated than plantar flexion if it is minimal. Too much dorsiflexion at the ankle results in a painful, uncomfortable heel strike and unsatisfactory push-off power. In determining ankle dorsiflexion during hindfoot and ankle reconstruction with medullary fixation, the surgeon must take into account forefoot equinus (**Fig. 6**).[37]

Gellman and colleagues[38] determined that the deficits after ankle fusion alone were 51% and 70%, respectively, for dorsiflexion and plantar flexion. Deficits in dorsiflexion and plantar flexion are 53% and 71%, respectively, after tibiotalocalcaneal fusion and were not significantly different from the deficits after ankle fusion alone. These authors found that inversion and eversion, however, were 40% less after tibiotalocalcaneal fusion than after ankle fusion alone. Deficits after pantalar arthrodesis were significant.

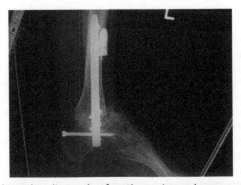

Fig. 5. Postoperative lateral radiograph of patient pictured preoperatively in **Fig. 2** after tibiotalocalcaneal arthrodesis with tibiotalar dorsiflexion osteotomy, debridement of dysvascular talar bone, and medullary nail fixation.

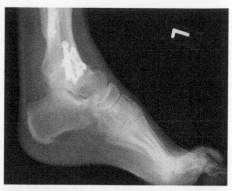

Fig. 6. Lateral radiograph of 60-year-old man who underwent dorsiflexion tibiotalar arthrodesis for posttraumatic ankle osteoarthritis, taking into account his recalcitrant forefoot equinus. Note that his hindfoot is fused in slight dorsiflexion to accommodate his forefoot equinus and transverse tarsal joint motion.

In dorsiflexion and plantar flexion, they were 63% and 82%, respectively. Inversion and eversion were 72% and 67% less, respectively, after pantalar arthrodesis than they were after ankle fusion alone.[38]

A patient's longitudinal biomechanical axis must be such that weight-bearing forces are carried directly through the center of the hip, knee, and ankle. It is normal that the heel be in approximately 5° of valgus and to the lateral side of that line.[9,39] Another general principle is that the surgeon should fuse all painful or arthritic joints but use joint-sparing procedures, such as cheilectomy and periarticular realignment osteotomies, whenever possible. When the surgeon does perform arthrodesis, the fusion should be fixed as rigidly as possible, the bone should be grafted liberally, and the fusion should be protected postoperatively. Bony prominences should be resected or osteotomized off the plantar weight-bearing aspect of the foot. Hardware and bone prominences should not be left in subcutaneous places of prominence, such as the retrocalcaneum.

The surgeon should avoid the formation of painful scars and neuromas, transposing the latter whenever they are encountered. In short, the surgeon should use a no-touch technique and be gentle with the soft tissues. Fascia and dermal tissues should be closed well so that the skin edges may be apposed and everted without tension at the end of the case. Along these lines, the surgeon should also preserve the plantar padding and stage procedures on different days when the magnitude of the deformity necessitates. For example, a patient with pantalar arthritis might be better served with a healthy, well-aligned triple arthrodesis of the hindfoot and a total ankle replacement above it than with a pantalar fusion using intramedullary fixation devices.[8]

Intramedullary nailing has proved to be a solid method of fixation for achieving ankle and hindfoot arthrodesis.[16,19,25] A nail inserted through the plantar aspect of the foot can afford excellent stability, position, and alignment. The process of ankle and hindfoot arthrodesis, often called tibiotalocalcaneal arthrodesis, uses an intramedullary nail and usually involves an ankle arthrotomy, preparation of the joint surfaces, and placement of the nail through a plantar incision. Screws are placed proximally through the tibia and the nail in a standard fashion. After compression across the fusion sites, the nail can be mechanically locked distally with screws into the calcaneus and talus.[5]

In a patient with severe external rotational deformity of the foot on the leg or a patient who has severe preoperative valgus deformity with the apex directed medially, the author usually positions the patient supine on the operating room table. The foot is positioned with the heel close to the end of a radiolucent operating room table with C-arm intraoperative fluoroscopic imaging available. A note is made of the anatomy of the contralateral uninvolved lower extremity and the mechanical axis of the index extremity. Most patients have adequate external rotation and internal rotation at the hip to allow anteroposterior and lateral imaging of the foot intraoperatively with the fluoroscope. For medullary nail fixation devices that allow for multiplanar locking screws to be inserted, even the supine patient—given enough flexion and rotation at the hip—can be managed appropriately in this fashion. General or regional anesthesia is used. Regional blocks for postoperative pain relief are used on a regular basis in the author's practice. Parenteral antibiotics are given on a prophylactic basis preoperatively. Landmarks are noted and the skin incision is designed to minimize soft tissue trauma and stripping.

Under thigh tourniquet hemostatic control, a longitudinal incision is usually made over the apex of the deformity medially in a patient with preoperative valgus. Dissection is carried sharply through the dermis, and blunt dissection is used deep to that exposing the medial malleolus in this approach. Care is taken to note and protect the course of the posterior tibial tendon and the posteromedial neurovascular bundle.

The patient with severe preoperative valgus generally undergoes a medial malleolar osteotomy to include a varus-producing, medially based closing wedge osteotomy through the tibiotalar fusion site (**Fig. 7**). If the subtalar joint is also in severe valgus, a small sinus tarsi incision can be made to approach the subtalar joint from the lateral side translating it medially and leaving it such that the calcaneus lines in collinear fashion with the talus and tibia. Alternatively, a careful medial approach to the subtalar joint can be made just dorsal to the posterior tibial tendon and posteromedial to the neurovascular bundle. This medial approach in patients who present with severe

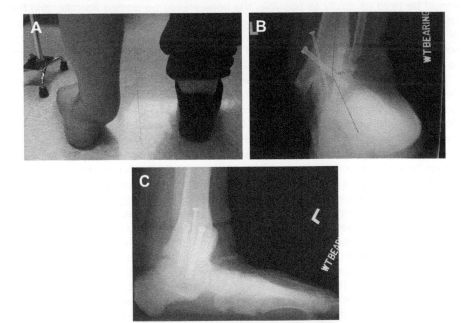

Fig. 7. Preoperative weight-bearing clinical appearance (A), anteroposterior radiograph (B), and lateral radiograph (C) of an obese 69-year-old man after valgus nonunion of attempted tibiotalar arthrodesis.

preoperative valgus obviates the potential problem of closing a lateral wound under tension once the valgus has been corrected.

Chisel, curette, and rongeur are used to denude diseased articular cartilage. Multiple fenestrations are made with a small-diameter drill bit on either side of the arthrodesis site to perforate hard subchondral bone and encourage bleeding and bony ingrowth. Once a collinear reduction of the tibia, talus, and calcaneus is achieved, a small plantar incision is made longitudinally anterior to the subcalcaneal fat pad. Sharp dissection is carried through the dermis with blunt dissection taken deep to that. A blunt key elevator is used to sweep away the intrinsic muscles and neurovascular structures on the plantar aspect of the foot. In this fashion, blunt dissection can be taken all the way down to the inferior surface of the calcaneus. The ideal starting point for the insertion of a guidewire is approximately 2 cm proximal to the calcaneal cuboid joint and lateral to the sustentaculum tali.

In this fashion, a guidewire is passed through the inferior cortex of the calcaneus, across the subtalar and ankle fusion sites, and into the distal tibia. Its position is ascertained on the anteroposterior and lateral projections of the C-arm fluoroscopic image and overdrilled with a cannulated drill bit measuring approximately 7 mm in diameter. The drill and its guidewire are removed and a bulb-tipped guidewire is passed in retrograde fashion through the calcaneus and talus and into the medullary canal of the distal tibia. A series of progressively larger flexible reamers are passed over this bulb-tipped guidewire to prepare the tibiotalocalcaneal canal for the nail. We usually start with an end-cutting reamer of approximately 8 mm in diameter then ream in half-millimeter increments up to 0.5 to 1.0 mm larger than the intended outside diameter of the nail to be used for fixation. A more aggressive advance in the width of the reamers can result in incarceration of the reamer within the tibia.

The length of the nail chosen should be such that its proximal tip does not end at the distal metadiaphyseal tibial isthmus. Overzealous reaming or the presence of a titanium medullary nail can cause a potential stress riser leading to cortical stress hypertrophy and insufficiency fractures. Ideally, a 15- to 18-cm nail can be inserted in retrograde fashion and end either distal or just proximal to this isthmus. In neuropathic patients, nails as long as 270 to 300 mm have been used to provide better stability and off-load stresses of the neuroarthropathic hindfoot.

As a general rule, it is critical to span skeletal defects, including those left by removal of hardware placed at prior procedures, by at least 1.5 to 2 tibial diameters. Failure to do so results in a stress riser and potential fracture through the defect. The distal end of the nail should be countersunk or flush with the inferior cortex of the calcaneus. Most manufacturers' nails include the capability of compression across the ankle and subtalar fusion sites, and the surgeon usually does best by countersinking the nail into the hindfoot to the depth he or she anticipates will compress across the fusion sites to prevent prominence.

The nail is locked proximally in the tibia with at least two locking screws that can be targeted with extramedullary aiming devices or freehanded for the longer, more proximal nails.It is advantageous to add bone graft across the fusion sites before inserting the nail and compressing the arthrodesis site. Compression across the ankle fusion site is often improved by osteotomizing the lateral malleolus if the fibula is intact. At this point it is imperative to check the rotation of the limb before locking distally. Ideally, the ankle should be in 0° of dorsiflexion and no more than 5° to 7° of hindfoot valgus, and it should have external rotation either symmetric with the contralateral uninvolved side or in a position at which the second ray of the foot lines up with the anteromedial tibial crest of the involved leg.

The nail is then locked distally in the talus and calcaneus (**Fig. 8**). I have found it advantageous to have a nail with multiplanar locking choices. Bench studies have documented as much as 40% increase in torsional rigidity when locking screws are placed at orthogonal angles.[5] Recent advances in medullary nail techniques include targeting slots for placement of tangential fixation screws from the calcaneus into the distal tibia. This use of a screw spanning the subtalar and tibiotalar joints can greatly increase the torsional rigidity of the construct and augments the fixation in the talus and calcaneus.[12] Often when one addresses the preoperative valgus deformity such as described here, it is impossible to lock distally from medial to lateral without putting at risk the medial neurovascular structures. If this is the case, lateral-to-medial and posterior-to-anterior locking screws are used for distal fixation. Further bone grafting is done and, if indicated, implanted bone stimulation devices are inserted. I have found it helpful to add demineralized bone matrix putty at the fusion sites to increase healing rates and help with hemostasis. An end cap is placed on the nail after its targeting device is removed to restrict medullary blood flow and protect the threads of the nail in the event that its removal be required in the future. Most nails are not inserted with the intention of removal and may be left in place indefinitely.

Locking screw heads are countersunk wherever possible so they are not prominent subcutaneously. The wound is usually closed over a closed suction drainage tube and a bulky dressing incorporating posterior and coaptation plaster splints applied with gentle compression wrap over padding. The drain is placed to suction and the patient is brought to the recovery area after checking circulatory status, position, and

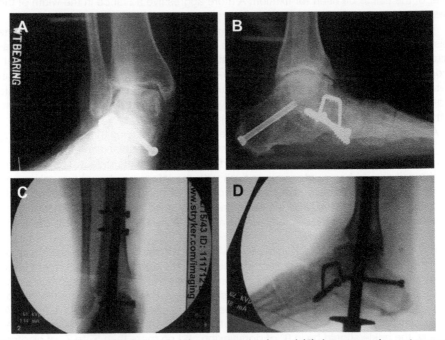

Fig. 8. Preoperative anteroposterior (*A*), preoperative lateral (*B*), intraoperative anteroposterior (*C*), and intraoperative lateral (*D*) radiographs of a 76-year-old woman who underwent pantalar arthrodesis with a medullary nail after triple arthrodesis for grade IV posterior tibial tendon insufficiency and ankle arthritis.

alignment. Permanent radiographs are helpful, and plantigrade reduction must be confirmed on the table before the patient's anesthesia is reversed. The surgeon must ensure satisfactory alignment, reduction, position, and fixation before terminating the case.

The patient with preoperative varus deformity or instability and weakness is positioned in the lateral decubitus position with the affected side up. A radiolucent operating room table is used and an axillary roll is used in the recumbent axilla. Great care is taken to pad all bony prominences, and the patient is fastened to the table with the contralateral limb flexed at the hip and knee so as to be out of the way for fluoroscopic imaging. The patient with good external rotation at the hip is afforded appropriate fluoroscopic imaging without having to rotate the C-arm. For the patient with severe preoperative varus, I would choose the transfibular approach, which affords excellent exposure for ankle and subtalar fusion (see **Fig. 1**).[4,5,13,40,41] The patient's own fibula also serves as a wonderful source of autogenous bone graft material. The patient undergoing medullary fixation for this type of preoperative deformity also has better shoe fit without impingement of a prominent fibula using the transfibular approach.

A longitudinal incision is made over the posterior fibula, which then curves anteriorly at its distal tip along the peroneal tendons. Care is taken to note the course of the existing neurovascular structures and tendons. The distal 4 to 5 cm of fibula is resected in a beveled fashion at a level approximately 2 cm proximal to the tibiotalar joint line, which normally preserves the distal tibiofibular syndesmosis and postoperatively prevents fibular instability (**Fig. 9**). Alternatively, the distal fibula can be skeletonized, osteotomized, and later re-fixated with screws to the tibia and talus to add to the fusion mass.[25]

The peroneal tendons are preserved, as is the thick periosteal envelope from which the fibula was harvested. This is saved to be used as a discreet anatomic layer for closure at the end of the case. An incision is extended distally to the sinus tarsi to allow subtalar joint visualization. Ankle and subtalar joint preparation are crucial to

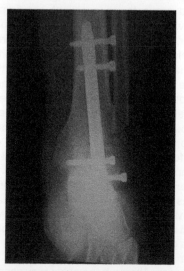

Fig. 9. Anteroposterior postoperative radiograph of patient pictured in **Fig. 1** after undergoing left tibiotalocalcaneal realignment and arthrodesis using transfibular approach.

successful fusion, and the author uses chisels, curettes, and rongeurs and multiple holes for fenestration. The tibiotalar joint can be denuded of cartilage in a congruent fashion to preserve the normal distal tibial concavity and talar dome convexity. In this fashion, external rotation positioning is easier to ascertain.

Alternatively, a transverse saw cut can be made across the distal tibia and the dome of the talus to bring the ankle into neutral position as the matching talar cut is performed.[13] The posterior and lateral talar surfaces are decorticated to allow for greater fusion surface, and the articular surface of the medial malleolus is denuded of diseased cartilage. The best position for arthrodesis is neutral dorsiflexion and approximately 5° of hindfoot valgus with external rotation symmetric with contralateral uninvolved extremity. Appropriate external rotation is achieved when the anteromedial crest of the tibia lies parallel to the second ray of the involved foot.[34,37] After preparation of the bony surfaces, a 2- to 3-cm longitudinal plantar incision is made anterior to the subcalcaneal fat pad.

The ideal position for the plantar calcaneal entry site is well anterior to the weight-bearing surface of the calcaneal tuberosity and approximately 2 cm posterior to the articulation of the calcaneus with the transverse tarsal joints. In the coronal plane, the entry site should line up with the center of the tibial medullary canal. Guidewires and flexible reamers are used to prepare the tibiotalocalcaneal canal.[7]

Once inserted, the proximal end of the nail should extend at least 1.5 to 2 tibial diameters above any potential cortical stress risers, including nonunion sites, tibial fractures, osteotomies sites, or cortical holes that may exist after previous hardware removal. Ideally the nail should be countersunk 5 to 10 mm in the plantar cortex of the calcaneus. In certain cases of tibiocalcaneal fusion, it is not unusual to have the distal portion of the nail extend 5 to 10 mm distal to the inferior cortex of the calcaneus and still have a sufficient plantar pad for pain-free weight bearing postoperatively. The remainder of the outrigger assembly targeting nail insertion and locking with compression across the fusion sites is as described previously.[5]

The techniques previously described appropriately address most patients who present with deformities ranging from the extremes of varus to valgus hindfoot malalignment in the coronal plane and any axial malalignment in the transverse plane. The patients described would prove to be excellent candidates for tibiotalocalcaneal arthrodesis. Patients for whom there is fixed deformity, including and distal to the transverse joints, however, must be considered for additional surgical procedures. It is imperative that the forefoot be plantigrade in such a fashion that the first and fifth metatarsals head strike the ground with weight bearing at the same time.

The patient with severe preoperative pes planovalgus and a fixed forefoot varus requires either derotational osteotomies through the transverse tarsal joints to a plantigrade posture and extension of the fusion mass to include a pantalar arthrodesis with medullary nail fixation (see **Fig. 8**) or, if the transverse tarsal joints are not arthritic, a plantar flexion opening wedge osteotomy at the base of the first metatarsal or through the medial cuneiform. In this fashion, the patient's first and fifth metatarsal heads strike the ground appropriately.[3,5,12]

The patient with preoperative pes cavovarus and fixed forefoot valgus presents the opposite problem and has a hyperplantarflexed first ray that requires either pantalar arthrodesis or, if the transverse tarsal joints are to be preserved, a dorsiflexion osteotomy at the base of the first metatarsal in order to achieve a plantigrade posture.[3,5,12,33] Fixed forefoot equinus, as often happens in the patient with pes cavus, must be taken into account when determining the appropriate position of hindfoot and ankle fusion with medullary fixation devices. Although the ankle may seem as if it is at neutral dorsiflexion relative to the long axis of the tibia, if the surgeon does not account for the fixed preoperative forefoot equinus, the patient still walks postoperatively with a back-kneed, recurvatum-type gait.[38] To preserve midfoot and forefoot mobility when addressing such patients, I often perform an anterior, closing wedge dorsiflexion osteotomy through the tibiotalar fusion site before fixing it with a medullary fixation device to ensure a plantigrade posture postoperatively (see **Fig. 2**).

AFTERCARE

In the author's personal series of using medullary fixation for hindfoot and ankle reconstruction, more than 95% union rate occurred within 12 to 14 weeks after surgery for patients undergoing the index fusion for diagnoses of osteoarthritis or rheumatoid arthritis. I prefer that the patient be immobilized in a non–weight-bearing, short-leg cast for the first 6 weeks followed by weight bearing to tolerance in a walking cast for an additional 6 weeks. Often transition to regular shoes is aided by the use of a removable fracture orthosis that includes a rocker bottom. I prefer to immobilize the neuropathic patients at least 4 weeks longer than the 12-week routine previously mentioned. Radiographs are obtained intraoperatively with suture removal 2 weeks postoperatively and every 4 weeks until union. Radiographs are obtained in the anteroposterior and lateral projection on a cassette long enough to include the entire length of a medullary nail.

SUMMARY

Medullary nail fixation for reconstruction of multiplanar, ankle, and hindfoot deformities has proven a safe, effective, and reliable method of fixation. The best results in achieving arthrodesis with this method are achieved for patients undergoing their index reconstruction procedure for a diagnosis of primary osteoarthritis or rheumatoid arthritis. Close attention to preoperative planning and intraoperative detail ensures the best possible outcomes with fewest complications.

REFERENCES

1. Ansart MB. Pan-arthrodesis for paralytic flail foot. J Bone Joint Surg 1951;33(B): 503–7.
2. Davis RJ, Mills MB. Ankle arthrodesis in the management of traumatic ankle arthrosis: a long-term retrospective study. J Trauma 1980;20:674–8.
3. Papa J, Myerson M, Girard P. Salvage, with arthrodesis, in intractable diabetic neuropathic arthropathy of the foot and ankle. J Bone Joint Surg Am 1993;75: 1056–66.
4. Iwata H, Yasuhara N, Kawashima K, et al. Arthrodesis of the ankle joint with rheumatoid arthritis: experience with the transfibular approach. Clin Orthop 1980;153: 189–93.
5. Quill GE. Tibiotalocalcaneal and pantalar arthrodesis. Foot Ankle Clin 1996;1(1): 199–210.
6. Kitaoka HB. Salvage of nonunion following ankle arthrodesis for failed total ankle arthroplasty. Clin Orthop Relat Res 1991;268:37–43.
7. Quill GE. Tibiotalocalcaneal arthrodesis. Tech Orthop 1996;11(3):269–73.
8. Quill GE. Triple arthrodesis of the foot with autogenous bone grafting: surgery videotape library. Rosemont (IL): American Academy of Orthopaedic Surgeons; 1995.
9. Quill GE. Subtalar arthrodesis. In: Myerson M, editor. Current therapy in foot and ankle surgery. Chicago: Mosby-Yearbook; 1993. p. 100–4.

10. Barrett GR, Meyer LC, Bray EW, et al. Pantalar arthrodesis: a long-term follow-up. Foot Ankle 1981;1:279–83.
11. Hamsa WR. Panastragaloid arthrodesis. J Bone Joint Surg Am 1935;18:732–6.
12. Papa JA, Myerson MS. Pantalar and tibiotalocalcaneal arthrodesis for post-traumatic osteoarthrosis of the ankle and hindfoot. J Bone Joint Surg Am 1992;74: 1042–9.
13. Miller SD, Myerson MS. Tibiotalar arthrodesis. In: Myerson MS, editor, Foot and Ankle Clinics, vol. 1. Philadelphia: WB Saunders; 1996. p. 151–62.
14. Cierney G, Cook G, Mader J. Ankle arthrodesis in the presence of ongoing sepsis. Orthop Clin North Am 1989;20:709–21.
15. Holt RS, Hansen ST, Mayo KA, et al. Ankle arthrodesis using internal screw fixation. Clin Orthop Relat Res 1991;268:21–8.
16. Küntscher G. Combined arthrodesis of the ankle and subtalar joints. In: Practice of intramedullary nailing. Springfield (IL): Charles C Thomas; 1967. p. 207–9.
17. Casadel R, Ruggierl P, Guiseppe T, et al. Ankle resection arthrodesis in patients with bone tumors. Foot Ankle Int 1994;15:242–9.
18. Boyd HB. Indications for fusion of the ankle. Orthop Clin North Am 1974;5(1): 191–2.
19. Carrier DA, Harris CM. Ankle arthrodesis with vertical Steinmann's pins in rheumatoid arthritis. Clin Orthop Relat Res 1991;268:10–4.
20. Cracchiolo AC. Methods and follow-up statistics on ankle arthrodesis. Clin Orthop Relat Res 1991;268:2–111.
21. Gilberson RG, Janes JM. Tibiocalcaneal fusion: a surgical technique. Surg Gynecol Obstet 1954;99:773–6.
22. Gruen GS, Mears DC. Arthrodesis of the ankle and subtalar joints. Clin Orthop Relat Res 1991;268:15–20.
23. Hunt WS, Thompson HA. Pantalar arthrodesis: a one-stage operation. J Bone Joint Surg Am 1954;36:349–63.
24. Reckling FW. Early tibiotalocalcaneal fusion in the treatment of severe injuries of the talus. J Trauma 1972;12:390–6.
25. Bingold AC. Ankle and subtalar fusion by a transarticular graft. J Bone Joint Surg Br 1956;38:862–70.
26. Charnley J. Compression arthrodesis of the ankle and shoulder. J Bone Joint Surg Br 1951;33:180–91.
27. Marek FM, Schein AJ. Aseptic necrosis of the astragalus following arthrodesing procedures of the talus. J Bone Joint Surg Am 1945;27:587–94.
28. Russotti GM, Johnson KA, Cass JR. Tibiotalocalcaneal arthrodesis for arthritis and deformity of the hind part of the foot. J Bone Joint Surg 1988;70(A):1304–7.
29. Soren A, Waugh TR. The historical evolution of arthrodesis of the foot. Int Orthop 1980;4:3–11.
30. Staples OS. Posterior arthrodesis of the ankle and subtalar joints. J Bone Joint Surg Am 1956;38(1):50–8.
31. Steindler A. The treatment of the flail ankle: panastragaloid arthrodesis. J Bone Joint Surg Am 1923;5:284–94.
32. Stuart MJ, Morrey BF. Arthrodesis of the diabetic neuropathic ankle. Clin Orthop 1990;253:209–11.
33. Vahvanen V. Arthrodesis of the TC or pantalar joints in rheumatoid arthritis. Acta Orthop Scand 1969;40:642–52.
34. Hefu FL, Baumann JU, Morscher EW. Ankle joint fusion: determination of optimal position by gait analysis. Arch Orthop Trauma Surg 1980;96:187–95.

35. Jackson A, Glasgow M. Tarsal hypermobility after ankle fusion: fact or fiction? J Bone Joint Surg Am 1979;61:470.
36. Mann RA. Biomechanics of the foot and ankle. In: Mann RA, Coughlin MJ, editors. Surgery of the foot and ankle. 6th edition. Chicago: Mosby; 1993. p. 28–32.
37. King HA, Watkins TB Jr, Samuelson KM. Analysis of foot position in ankle arthrodesis and its influence on gait. Foot Ankle 1980;1:44–9.
38. Gellman H, Lenihan M, Halikis N, et al. Selective tarsal arthrodesis: an in-vitro analysis of the effect on foot motion. Foot Ankle 1987;8:127–33.
39. Inman TV. The subtalar joint. In: Inman TV, editor. The joints of the ankle. Baltimore (MD): Williams & Wilkins; 1976. p. 37.
40. Adams JC. Arthrodesis of the ankle joint: experiences with the transfibular approach. J Bone Joint Surg 1948;30B:506–11.
41. Horwitz T. The use of the transfibular approach in arthrodesis of the ankle joint. Am J Surg 1942;55:550–2.

The Indications and Technique of Supramalleolar Osteotomy

Adam S. Becker, MD[a,b], Mark S. Myerson, MD[a,]*

KEYWORDS

• Deformity • Distal tibia • Ankle arthritis • Reconstruction

The supramalleolar osteotomy is a commonly used surgical procedure to correct congenital or acquired deformities of the distal tibia, ankle, or foot. In children, osteotomy has been used to correct malunion of fractures, physeal growth arrest, tibial torsion, paralytic deformities, and sequelae of a clubfoot.[1–8] More recently, distal tibial osteotomies are being used to correct lower extremity, ankle and foot deformities in adults to prolong ankle function and avoid the need for an ankle arthrodesis. The goal of these procedures is to realign the limb in the setting of these deformities and to redistribute the loads on the ankle joint, thereby improving the biomechanics of the lower extremity.[9] The same premise applies to the use of osteotomies as a treatment alternative for ankle arthritis.[10,11] This article focuses on the current indications, the technique, and different modes of fixation for supramalleolar osteotomies.

BIOMECHANICS OF DEFORMITY CORRECTION

The relationship between deformity and ankle arthrosis is not clear, as there is no clear consensus regarding the tolerated limits of angular deformity of the tibia and the potential for development of ankle arthritis. Laboratory models that simulate distal tibial deformities have demonstrated the changes in contact pressures within the tibiotalar joint that occur with deformity. Tarr and colleagues established that distal deformities with angulation of 15° showed up to a 42% reduction in contact area, with

---

Dr. Myerson is a consultant for DePuy Orthopedics (Warsaw, Indiana), Biomet (Parsipinnay, New Jersey), and Orthohelix (Akron, Ohio). He receives royalties on products that may be discussed in this article.

[a] Institute for Foot and Ankle Reconstruction, Mercy Medical Center, 301 St. Paul Place, Baltimore, MD 21202, USA
[b] Englewood Orthopedic Associates, 401 South Van Brunt Street, Englewood, NJ 07631, USA
* Corresponding author.
E-mail address: mark4feet@aol.com (M.S. Myerson).

Foot Ankle Clin N Am 14 (2009) 549–561
doi:10.1016/j.fcl.2009.06.002

foot.theclinics.com

greater changes observed with sagittal plane deformities. In addition, this study also revealed that limitation of subtalar motion decreased ankle contact area, emphasizing the importance of the compensatory role of the subtalar joint with a tibial deformity.[9] Cooper and colleagues[12] confirmed this finding by showing that a 10° valgus supramalleolar osteotomy decreased the force on the medial talar dome by 42%. Kristensen and colleagues,[13,14] however, reported on 22 patients who had tibia fractures with more than 10° of angular malunion at 20 years after the injury. Thirty-eight percent were asymptomatic, and no patients had limitations of ankle motion greater than 10° or radiographic signs of ankle arthrosis. The ability of the ankle and foot to tolerate deformity above the ankle depends on the flexibility and the ability of the foot to accommodate and compensate for the deformity. With a distal tibia varus or valgus deformity, the subtalar joint must evert or invert to maintain a plantigrade forefoot, which is compromised if the hindfoot is stiff. The clinical examination of the foot is therefore important to plan for the correction of a distal tibia deformity. In general, the authors have found that valgus deformity of the distal tibia or ankle is tolerated better than varus, largely because of the ability of the subtalar joint, which can invert far more than evert.[15,16] It is likely from that a 10° valgus distal tibial deformity can be compensated for by the foot, but this ultimately may be associated with abnormal ankle biomechanics and arthrosis. Generally, the authors recommend correcting deformity greater than 10° in any plane, which will change if the hindfoot is stiff.

INDICATIONS FOR OSTEOTOMY

A supramalleolar osteotomy is indicated to address deformity at, above, or below the ankle joint, and ankle arthrosis associated with intra-articular varus or valgus deformity. Multiplanar distal tibial deformity with angular and translational components alters the weight-bearing axis of the tibia through the ankle joint. In these patients, an osteotomy can be used to correct the malalignment and to prevent the development of degenerative changes, or in cases with ankle arthritis, to alter joint mechanics and shift loads onto intact articular cartilage. Correction of malunion through an ankle fusion is accomplished easier through a distal tibial osteotomy, as residual equinus leads to lengthening of the extremity and recurvatum thrust at the knee, and increases stresses in the midfoot. Dorsiflexion malunion of an ankle fusion results in increased stress seen in the heel pad at heel strike. Varus and valgus malunions lead to overload of the lateral and medial columns, respectively, in addition to resulting in a stiff transverse tarsal joint and excessive flatfoot. Many cases of ankle arthrosis that otherwise would be candidates for a total ankle arthroplasty are complicated by distal tibial malalignment that would lead to early failure of the arthroplasty. Correction and balancing of the lower leg mechanical axis through a distal tibial osteotomy as a staging procedure are necessities before ankle arthroplasty. In addition, distal tibial osteotomies can be used to correct deformities such as the fixed valgus deformity associated with a ball-in-socket ankle and deformities secondary to growth plate injury and neuropathy. The goal of treatment is to maintain the weight-bearing axis of the lower extremity centered over the ankle and subtalar joints. Supramalleolar osteotomy is also a very useful adjunct to the correction of an intra-articular varus deformity associated either with recurrent ankle instability or congenital distal tibia vara.

SURGICAL PLANNING

Surgical planning begins with physical examination of the patient. Examining a patient while he or she is standing can allow for evaluation for limb length discrepancy, pelvic obliquity, and heel or knee varus or valgus. Range of motion (ROM) testing of the ankle and subtalar joints is also very important. Limited ankle ROM can be secondary to gastrocnemius or *Achilles* contractures that can both addressed at the time of surgery. Adequate subtalar motion is needed to compensate for the supramalleolar correction of ankle coronal plane deformities. In normal feet, there is considerably more inversion than eversion, and therefore the hindfoot can compensate better for valgus-producing osteotomies. The skin and soft tissues surrounding the distal tibia and ankle need to be evaluated carefully. One of the most significant complications of a supramalleolar osteotomy is related to wound healing or soft tissue compromise. In most patients, there will be previous scars or soft tissue flaps present in the peri-articular area, which will influence one's decision on surgical approach and technique. The magnitude of correction and the possible lengthening of long standing deformities can place surrounding soft tissue under increased tension, leading to subsequent wound complications.

The normal anatomic relationships of the leg and ankle must be understood before attempting a distal tibial osteotomy. The mechanical (anatomic) axis of the distal tibia is the extension of the mechanical axis of the lower extremity. The mechanical axis distally extends through the center of the ankle joint. The tibial plafond on the antero-posterior (AP) radiographic view forms an angle of 93° with the mechanical axis of the tibia called the distal tibial ankle surface angle (TAS). On the lateral radiograph, this angle is referred to as the tibial lateral surface angle (TLS), normal averaging 80° **(Fig. 1)**.[17,18] When performing a distal osteotomy, the surgeon's goal should be to restore the TAS and TLS back to within normal values when compared with the contra-lateral limb and perhaps even overcorrection slightly to anticipate some collapse through the osteotomy site. Planning of the extremity correction starts with full-length radiographs of the bilateral lower extremities. Limb lengths and the overall mechanical axis are measured along with the respected articular angles. If leg length inequality is present, then performing an opening wedge or dome osteotomy is performed, as a closing wedge osteotomy would lead to further shortening.

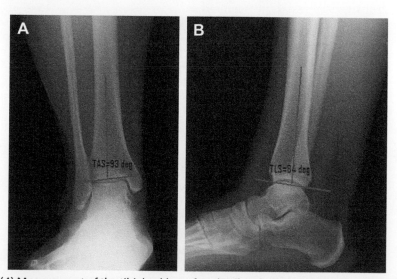

Fig. 1. (*A*) Measurement of the tibial ankle surface (TAS) and tibial lateral surface (TLS) angles on the AP and lateral radiographs in a normal patient. (*B*) The mechanical axis is drawn followed by the distal tibial angle on the respective radiographs.

Multiplanar deformities often involve coronal and sagittal components, which can result in a combination of ankle varus, valgus, recurvatum, procurvatum, translation, and rotation. The types of deformities are measured and described by the center of rotation and angulation (CORA). The CORA is created by intersecting the mechanical axis of the proximal and distal segments making up the deformity (**Fig. 2**). Care must be taken to evaluate the ankle joint for erosions of the tibial plafond or deformity through the ankle joint, as these too need to be addressed. When the corrective osteotomy is made at the level of the CORA, then the anatomy can be restored with angular and rotational correction without translation of the distal fragment. In such cases where the osteotomy needs to be made above or below the CORA, as in ankle arthrodesis malunion or impaction fractures of the tibial plafond, the distal segment will need to be translated relative to the mechanical axis. To avoid creating a secondary translational deformity distally, when the osteotomy is made at a different level than the CORA, the osteotomy line will to be translated.[19] For example, with a medial closing wedge osteotomy, the distal tibial fragment needs to be translated laterally to avoid a secondary medial translational deformity. In these cases of ankle deformities, correction needs to be performed well above the CORA to accommodate for rigid fixation.

SURGICAL TECHNIQUE

Distal tibial osteotomies are performed under general anesthesia, usually with a popliteal block for postoperative pain control. The approach is through a medial incision centered at the level of the planned osteotomy. Periosteal stripping and skin retraction is kept to a minimum. Depending on the location of the osteotomy in relation to the CORA, the need for translation, and the degree of deformity correction, an oblique fibular osteotomy may be necessary to allow adequate correction. This is performed through a separate lateral incision. This osteotomy allows translation, rotation, and correction of significant angulation.

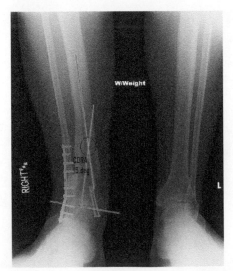

Fig. 2. Measurement of the center of rotation and angulation (CORA) is created by the intersection of the mechanical axis of both the proximal and distal segments making up the deformity.

CORRECTION OF VARUS DEFORMITY

Think about the cause of the deformity. Is the varus above or below the joint, or is it intra-articular? For each of these, a different approach is used, each performed with additional procedures as necessary to correct associated deformity. In fact, it is rare to perform an isolated tibial osteotomy, because these associated deformities necessitating correction are so common, and include ankle ligament reconstruction, calcaneus osteotomy, posterior and anterior tibial tendon transfer, hindfoot arthrodesis, first metatarsal osteotomy, and intra-articular procedures such as cheilectomy, arthroscopy, or ankle replacement. To correct the tibia, lengthening the medial column of the tibia or shortening of the lateral column of the tibia is necessary for correction. This can be accomplished by a medial opening wedge osteotomy, lateral closing wedge osteotomy, or a dome osteotomy (which the authors use commonly to correct multiplanar deformity). As a generalization, a medial opening wedge osteotomy almost always is used, because it is easier to perform; the healing and incorporation of the bone graft is good, and leg length can be restored or at least maintained. In distal tibial deformities where the CORA is at the level of the ankle joint, the tibial osteotomy is made 4 to 5 cm proximal to the tip of the medial malleolus, ideally remaining in metaphyseal bone. Through a medial incision, a k-wire is inserted under fluoroscopy and used as a cutting guide for a horizontal cut made using a wide oscillating saw, with care to leave the lateral cortex intact to act as a fulcrum. A periosteal elevator is inserted into the osteotomy site to distract slightly; this is replaced by a lamina spreader. Gentle distraction under fluoroscopy then is applied to the medial aspect of the osteotomy. The laminar spreader is opened gradually until the ankle joint line is parallel with the floor or perpendicular to the tibial axis. One has to be careful how the graft insertion is planned, because the laminar spreader may interfere with the insertion of the graft. One can use a distractor shaped like a lamina spreader without paddles and instead with pin holes in the side of the clamp (Integra, Plainsboro, New Jersey, USA), and the osteotomy can be distracted with the paddles of the laminar spreader preventing insertion of the graft. The bone graft wedge is cut to shape predetermined by preoperative calculations, and then inserted and tamped into place (**Fig. 3**). The authors always augment the allograft with an osteobiologic product, usually infiltrating the graft with a concentrate of mesenchymal cells obtained from an aspiration of the iliac crest. K-wires then are inserted to temporarily fix the osteotomy while internal fixation is applied. Single-plane, whether either coronal or sagittal, deformities usually are corrected fully with this technique; however, multiplanar deformities often require rotation and translation to attain full correction. For these multiplanar deformities, either a dome osteotomy is used, or a medial opening wedge osteotomy performed in the combined plane (coronal and sagittal). This is made under fluoroscopic guidance, not leaving the lateral cortex intact, allowing rotational and translational correction or with placement of an asymmetric structural allograft to maintain the alignment. There are indications for performing a closing lateral wedge osteotomy, although the authors do not use this procedure commonly (eg, when the medial skin is poor, where limb length is not of any importance, or where a lateral approach to correction is necessary in conjunction with additional ankle procedures).

CORRECTION OF VALGUS DEFORMITY

For valgus deformities, lengthening the lateral aspect of the tibia or shortening the medial aspect of the tibia is necessary. This can be accomplished using a closing medial wedge osteotomy, an opening lateral wedge osteotomy, or a dome osteotomy. A closing medial wedge osteotomy is preferred unless there is pre-existing shortening

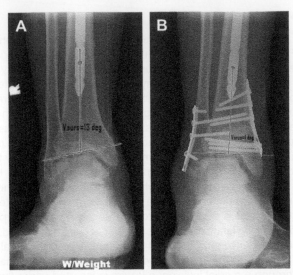

Fig. 3. Preoperative (A) and 2-year postoperative (B) radiographs of a patient with a 13° varus distal tibial alignment. After correction through a medial opening wedge osteotomy with an allograft wedge, the tibial ankle surface (TAS) was improved significantly.

of the limb. The base of the wedge is marked at the preoperatively planned level, and k-wires are placed under fluoroscopic guidance in a converging fashion at both proximal and distal aspects of the wedge meeting at the lateral cortex. The k-wires then are used as cutting guides, and the medial wedge is removed using a wide oscillating saw. Again, care is taken to leave the lateral periosteal sleeve intact to act as a fulcrum during deformity correction. Multiplanar deformities are corrected with either resection of an asymmetric wedge, or a closing wedge osteotomy in the combined plane of the deformity.

Multiplanar deformities of the distal tibia require meticulous preoperative planning, as they are more complex deformities. They are often the result of a combined varus, valgus deformities with rotational and translational components. Correction of these deformities requires angular as well as rotation and translation through the planned osteotomy. For these multiplanar deformities, an osteotomy in the combined deformity plane (coronal and sagittal) is made under fluoroscopic guidance, completing the osteotomy through both cortices. This allows rotational and translational correction through the osteotomy, correction by insertion of an asymmetric structural allograft, or resection of an asymmetric wedge to attain the planned correction.

A dome osteotomy is a useful technique that can be used to correct either varus or valgus deformities without the need to shorten the limb (**Fig. 4**). This osteotomy is done usually through an anterior lateral incision over the distal tibia. Care is taken to dissect and mobilize the neurovascular bundle and retract it away from the surgical field. The plane of the ankle joint is marked out using fluoroscopy by using a k-wire placed in a horizontal position parallel to the ankle joint. Using a 3.2 mm drill bit, multiple drill holes are created in the shape of a convex dome, with height of the dome approximately 1 to 1.5 cm. This could be done in a free-hand fashion or with the aide of Macquet drill guide. Care again is taken to remain within the metaphyseal bone of the distal tibia. Next, a fibular osteotomy is made at the same level. A 4 mm pin then is inserted into the distal tibial fragment parallel to the ankle joint, and a second pin is inserted into the tibial shaft 8 to 10 cm proximal to the osteotomy site. The

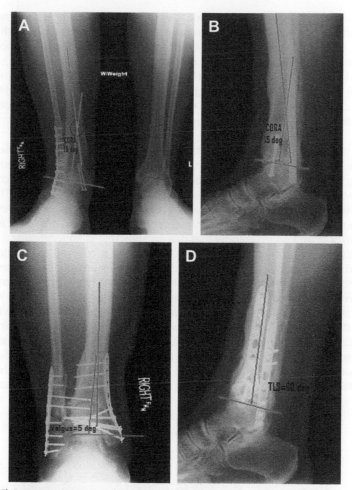

Fig. 4. (*A, B*) Preoperative AP and lateral radiographs (*top*) of 36-year-old man with distal malunion. (*C, D*) Correction of the deformity through a dome osteotomy (*bottom*) allowed sagittal, coronal, and rotational realignment.

osteotomy then is completed using an oscillating saw to connect the multiple drill holes. Correction of the frontal plane deformity is achieved by aligning the two 4 mm pins parallel to each other.

CORRECTION OF INTRA-ARTICULAR VARUS DEFORMITY

Ankle varus deformity may be associated with chronic ankle instability, and the deformity is usually intra-articular. The deformity is present both in the ankle and below it, because associated foot deformity is common. The ankle is usually quite unstable, and the heel in varus. Commonly, the peroneal tendons are torn, and the posterior and anterior tibial tendons are producing more varus deformity of the foot. The primary concern for these patients is whether an ankle arthrodesis can be avoided. Even with arthrodesis, the accompanying deformity must be corrected, and the foot well balanced with osteotomy and tendon transfer. The first objective is to establish whether the ankle is flexible or rigid, because the latter deformity is not amenable to the intra-articular osteotomy. The ankle is evaluated under fluoroscopy with a valgus producing stress manipulation. Once the talus has been reduced to a more lateral position, the intra-articular defect is more easily visible on the medial aspect of the joint as an indentation. This indentation in the joint line will persist following more traditional tibial osteotomy whether opening or closing wedge. For example, note in **Fig. 5** where the correction of the ankle varus was accomplished with a closing wedge distal tibia osteotomy, but the defect in the medial joint persisted, leading to recurrent varus deformity.

Even in the presence of ankle arthritis, realignment of the ankle with osteotomy is worthwhile, because the osteotomy will redistribute the forces on the medial ankle, prolonging the viability of a more normally aligned joint. A problem with the chronically unstable varus ankle is the dysplasia that occurs of the medial malleolus. The medial aspect of the malleolus is no longer vertical, and has a medially inclined articulation arising from chronic pressure of the medially driven talus. The only way to correct this deformity is with an osteotomy that has an apex that is intra-articular.

This unique intra-articular osteotomy of the plafond is referred to as the plafond-plasty, and it can correct varus and valgus deformities secondary to impaction injuries or chronic deformity of the plafond. The technique for the plafondplasty, is to first mark out the level and alignment of the distal tibia articular surface using a k-wire with intra-operative fluoroscopy. Then, a second k-wire is introduced parallel to the impacted portion of the tibial plafond. This second k-wire is inserted so the wire is within the subchondral bone just under the articular cartilage at the apex of the plafond angulation. This second k-wire then is used as a cutting guide to create an osteotomy, leaving the distal subchondral bone bridge intact. This bone bridge then is used as a hinge, and a wide osteotome is used to very gradually disimpact the plafond until the distal tibial

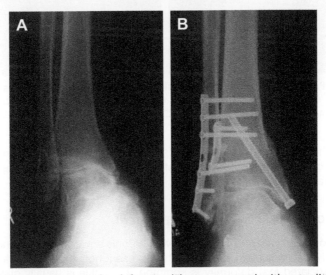

Fig. 5. (A) The varus intra-articular deformity (B) was corrected with a traditional closing wedge lateral tibial osteotomy. Although the weight-bearing forces were improved markedly with this procedure, the talus remains tilted, because the intra-articular medial distal tibial defect was not corrected. The medial malleolus remains tilted and dysplastic. The correction would have been better with an intra-articular osteotomy redirecting the orientation of the medial malleolus.

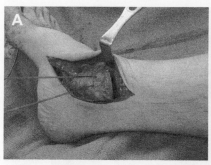
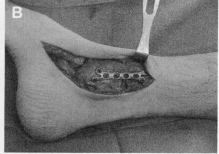

Fig. 6. The intraoperative photographs are presented, following the osteotomy and temporary fixation with k-wires (*A*), and then definitive fixation using an locking plate (*B*) (Orthohelix, Akron, Ohio).

articular surface is parallel to the intact portion of the distal tibia. A lamina spreader then is inserted into the cortical gap to hold the correction while bone graft is inserted into the defect created to maintain a parallel joint surface. A distal tibial plate (Orthohelix, Akron, Ohio) then is used for fixation to ensure the allograft remains in place and as support for the realigned plafond (**Fig. 6**). Care must be taken to insert the distal-most screws parallel to the joint to keep these screws extra-articular (**Figs. 7** and **8**).

Once the planning and execution of the distal tibial osteotomy are completed, the decision needs to be made on what type of fixation is needed. With the introduction of locking plate technology, surgeons now have a multitude of choices for fixation of osteotomies. The first decision is whether to use internal or external fixation. External fixation is necessary in complicated reconstructions that require gradual correction rather than acute one-stage corrections, or in cases of active infection.[19] In addition, if correction of a deformity that includes a significant limb length

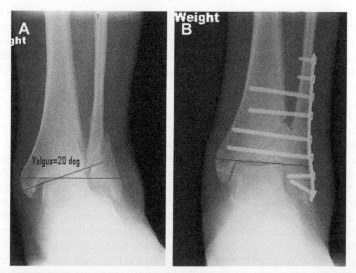

Fig. 7. Preoperative (*left*) (*A*) AP radiograph of 56-year-old man with 20° of lateral tibial plafond impaction. AP radiograph (*right*) (*B*) demonstrates correction of the impaction injury with lateral plafondplasty using an allograft wedge.

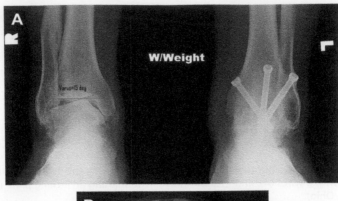

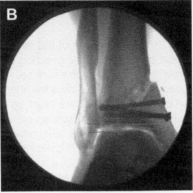

Fig. 8. Preoperative AP radiograph (*top*) (*A*) of varus malalignment after a distal tibia fracture with early arthritis of the medial ankle joint. Intraoperative radiograph (*bottom*) (*B*) with correction of ankle alignment and restoration of uniform ankle joint space.

discrepancy requires simultaneous lengthening through the osteotomy, then external fixation is the recommended method of fixation. Internal fixation has the advantages of acting as a buttress to hold the graft in place when performing an opening wedge osteotomy, being less cumbersome to patients, and having a lower risk of infection. With the introduction of locked plating technology, there are numerous options for internal fixations of distal tibial osteotomies. In metaphyseal bone such as the distal tibia, where fixation is sometimes more difficult or screw purchase is poor, fixation with locked plating has been shown to be biomechanically advantageous to conventional plating. Locked plating creates a single beam construct as a result of no movement allowed between the components of fixation such as the screws, plate, and bone. Single- beam constructs are four times stronger than load-sharing constructs, in which motion occurs between the individual fixation components. Locking plates act as internal fixed-angle devices, and as a result, they improve fixation where screw purchase may be inadequate. In addition, because the screws are at a fixed angle with the plate, all screws within the construct must fail simultaneously for the plate to pull off. There are various distal tibial locking plates on the market that are precontoured to the anatomy of the tibia, making percutaneous fixation easier and less invasive (**Fig. 9**).

Patients usually are placed in short-leg cast for the first 4 weeks and told not to put weight on the operated limb. At about 5 to 6 weeks, they are placed into a fracture boot, and ROM exercises without resistance are started. Initiating partial weight bearing depends on the stability of fixation and evidence of radiographic healing.

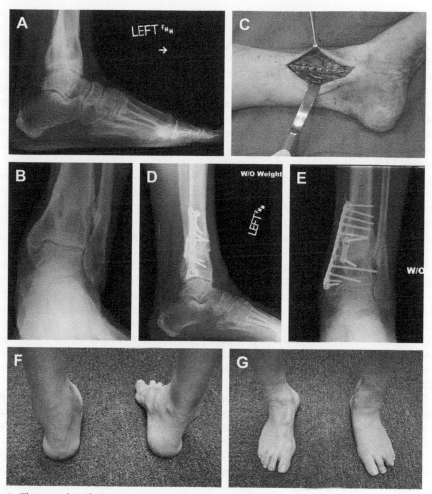

Fig. 9. The pre- (A, B), intraoperative (C), and postoperative x rays (D, E) and clinical align-ment (F, G) of a patient with severe post-traumatic deformity of the distal tibia. An opening wedge medial osteotomy was performed with rigid locking plate fixation (Orthohelix, Akron, Ohio). Note the realignment of the left leg following surgery.

OUTCOMES

Outcomes after supramalleolar osteotomies have been encouraging. The earliest long-term follow-up study by Takakura was of 18 patients, with an average of 7 years follow-up. Patients were treated with an anterior medial opening wedge osteotomy to correct a varus ankle deformity. Six patients had excellent results; nine had a good result, and three had fair result. The three patients who had fair results were most likely secondary to undercorrection of the deformity. Ten of the 18 patients had a second-look ankle arthroscopy that revealed 70% of patients showed evidence of fibrocartilage repair. Takakura in 1998 reported his results of medial opening wedge osteotomies for treating post-traumatic varus distal tibial deformities. Healing of the osteotomies was achieved at an average of 6 weeks, with one delayed union that healed at 6 months. His average preoperative TAS angle was 70°, and the postoperative average TAS angle was corrected to 87.1°. Six of the nine patients in this study complained of stiffness of the ankle postoperatively.[10,11]

Stamatis and colleagues published their results of using supramalleolar osteotomies for treating distal tibial deformities of at least 10° in patients who had ankle pain. Thirteen patients were treated, with an average follow-up of34 months. They showed improvements in American Orthopedic Foot and Ankle Society (AOFAS) scores from 54 to 87 points, and Takakura ankle scores improved from 57 to 82 points. The study showed correction of the valgus malalignment by measuring the average preoperative TAS angle of 107°, and the postoperative TAS angle corrected to an average of 92.6°. The correction of the varus deformities was from a preoperative average TAS angle of 72° to 86.6° postoperatively.[12]

Harstall and colleagues reported in 2007 on nine patients treated with lateral closing wedge osteotomies for varus ankle deformities. The average time to osseous union was 10 weeks. The average AOFAS scores improved from 48 to 74 points, and the average TAS angle improved from 6.9° of varus to 0.6° of valgus postoperatively. Two of the nine patients at final follow-up, however, showed radiographic progression of their ankle arthrosis.[20]

The use of a supramalleolar osteotomy for treating multiplanar deformities of the distal tibia has been reported by Graehl and colleagues. In this study, eight patients were presented who had distal tibial malunion with a mean varus angulation of 15°. All patients were treated with low tibial osteotomies. The investigators used dome osteotomies for coronal plane deformities and wedge osteotomies for biplanar and sagittal plane deformities. Seven out of eight patients improved significantly after their osteotomy. The investigators believe that adequate correction can be obtained by achieving maximum correction intraoperatively and by maintaining this correction with stable fixation.[21]

Complications with supramalleolar osteotomies are rare. The most common is stiffness of the ankle. Delayed union of these osteotomies is also rare; however, it has been reported in Takakura's and Stamatis' studies. In both studies, a total of three delayed unions occurred; however, all three healed by 6 months.

Clinical outcomes support the use of supramalleolar osteotomies as an effective surgical option for treating lower extremity deformities, whether congenital or posttraumatic. Meticulous preoperative planning of deformity correction and limb realignment helps redistribute joint forces safely and reliably within the ankle to prevent developing arthrosis or halting its progression.

REFERENCES

1. Abraham E, Lubicky JP, Songer MN, et al. Supramalleolar osteotomy for ankle valgus in myelomeningocele. J Pediatr Orthop 1996;16(6):774–81.
2. Malhotra D, Puri R, Owen R. Valgus deformity of the ankle in children with spina bifida aperta. J Bone Joint Surg Br 1984;66(3):381–5.
3. McNicol D, Leong JC, Hsu LC. Supramalleolar derotation osteotomy for lateral tibial torsion and associated equinovarus deformity of the foot. J Bone Joint Surg Br 1983;65(2):166–70.
4. Nicol RO, Menelaus MB. Correction of combined tibial torsion and valgus deformity of the foot. J Bone Joint Surg Br 1983;65(5):641–5.
5. Stevens PM, Otis S. Ankle valgus and clubfeet. J Pediatr Orthop 1999;19(4):515–7.
6. Coester LM, Saltzman CL, Leupold J, et al. Long-term results following ankle arthrodesis for post-traumatic arthritis. J Bone Joint Surg Am 2001;22:219–28.

7. Pyevich MT, Saltzman CL, Callaghan JJ, et al. Total ankle arthroplasty: a unique design. Two- to twelve-year follow-up. J Bone Joint Surg Am 1998;80(10): 1410–20.

8. Kumar SJ, Keret D, MacEwen GD. Corrective cosmetic supramalleolar osteotomy for valgus deformity of the ankle joint: a report of two cases. J Pediatr Orthop 1990;10(1):124–7.

9. Tarr RR, Resnick CT, Wagner KS, et al. Changes in tibiotalar joint contact areas following experimentally induced tibial angular deformities. Clin Orthop 1985; 199:72–80.

10. Takakura Y, Tanaka Y, Kumai T, et al. Low tibial osteotomy for osteoarthritis of the ankle. Results of a new operation in 18 patients. J Bone Joint Surg Br 1995;77(1): 50–4.

11. Takakura Y, Takaoka T, Tanaka Y, et al. Results of opening-wedge osteotomy for the treatment of a post-traumatic varus deformity of the ankle. J Bone Joint Surg Am 1998;80(2):213–8.

12. Stamatis ED, Cooper PS, Myerson MS. Supramalleolar osteotomy for the treatment of distal tibial angular deformities and arthritis of the ankle joint. Foot Ankle Int 2003;24(10):754–64.

13. Kristensen KD, Kiaer T, Blicher J. No arthrosis of the ankle 20 years after malaligned tibial shaft fracture. Acta Orthop Scand 1989;60(2):208–9.

14. Merchant TC, Dietz FR. Long-term follow-up after fractures of the tibial and fibular shafts. J Bone Joint Surg Am 1989;71(4):599–606.

15. Ting AJ, Tarr RR, Sarmiento A, et al. The role of subtalar motion and ankle contact pressure changes from angular deformities of the tibia. Foot Ankle 1987;7(5): 290–9.

16. Steffensmeier SJ, Saltzman CL, Berbaum KS, et al. Effects of medial and lateral displacement calcaneal osteotomies on tibiotalar joint contact stresses. J Orthop Res 1996;14(6):980–5.

17. Mangone PG. Distal tibial osteotomies for the treatment of foot and ankle disorders. Foot Ankle Clin 2001;6(3):583–97.

18. Egol KA, Kubiak EN, Fulkerson FJ, et al. Biomechanics of locked plates and screws. J Orthop Trauma 2004;18(8):488–93.

19. Paley D. The correction of complex foot deformities using Ilizarov's distraction osteotomies. Clin Orthop 1993;293:97–111.

20. Harstall R, Lehmann O, et al. Supramalleolar lateral closing wedge osteotomy for the treatment of varus ankle arthrosis. Foot Ankle Int 2007;28(5):542–8.

21. Gaehl PM, Hersh MR, Heckman JD, et al. Supramalleolar osteotomy for the treatment of symptomatic tibial malunion. J Orthop Trauma 1998;1:281.

Treatment of Nonunion and Malunion of Trauma of the Foot and Ankle Using External Fixation

Andrew Peter Molloy, MR, FRCS (Tr & Orth)[a],*, Andy Roche, MR, MRCS[a],
Badri Narayan, MR, FRCS (Tr & Orth)[b]

KEYWORDS

• External • Fixation • Nonunion • Malunion • Foot • Ankle

External fixation is a valuable clinical tool, because it allows the surgeon to promote healing of bone and correct deformities by static and dynamic means. External fixators are often quick and easy to apply and frequently suitable for damage control procedures in trauma scenarios. They have significant biologic advantages over internal fixation with preservation of tissue envelopes and blood supply. Therefore external fixators can be used in areas and occasions where internal fixation would pose a threat to wound healing and bone union. External fixation has its advantages over internal fixation, particularly where there is active infection in the foot or ankle, where methods of internal fixation almost certainly would succumb to infection.

Internal fixation can be problematic when utilized in areas with poor skin coverage, for example the distal tibia. This can predispose to either wound breakdown or symptoms secondary to prominence of the hardware through thin subcutaneous tissue. Incisions made for wide exposure for placement of internal fixation through poorly vascularized or edematous skin, often seen in diabetic patients, can predispose to wound breakdown and are therefore more amenable to percutaneous external fixation methods. Bone loss and paucity of bone quality are often problems in nonunion revision surgery, especially in the presence of infection or in patients who have Charcot joints. In these clinical scenarios, internal fixation becomes difficult, and the advantages of minimally invasive techniques in external fixation become apparent. The construction and versatility of fixators also afford the surgeon the ability to place the

[a] Department of Trauma and Orthopaedics, University Hospital Aintree, Lower Lane, Liverpool, L9 7AL, United Kingdom
[b] Department of Trauma and Orthopaedics, Royal Liverpool University Hospital, Prescot Street, Liverpool, L7 8XP, United Kingdom
* Corresponding author.
E-mail address: andy.molloy@aintree.nhs.uk (A.P. Molloy).

Foot Ankle Clin N Am 14 (2009) 563–587
doi:10.1016/j.fcl.2009.03.007
1083-7515/09/$ – see front matter © 2009 Elsevier Inc. All rights reserved.

foot.theclinics.com

percutaneous pins outside the zones of injury or arthrodesis, thus reducing the risk of vascular compromise and infection of the affected site. Although obviously safe corridors of passage of wires and pins have to be used, the ability to place them away from sites of previous surgery can prevent iatrogenic damage where scarring may have altered the normal course of the nerves. The construct of, especially circular, external fixators render sufficient inherent stability to allow early weight bearing and joint mobilization (in nonspanning fixators). This achieves early restoration of limb and joint function, one of the primary goals in any orthopedic intervention.

EXTERNAL FIXATOR CONSTRUCTS

External fixators used in modern orthopedics and trauma surgery encompass various constructs. The most basic are the mono-lateral fixators. The basic design is using threaded half pins connected by a rod (**Fig. 1**).

Stability depends on various factors. The bone–pin interface is the crux of stability, starting with a good hold and keeping a good hold of bone. Two important parameters that influence interface stresses and bone hold are pin diameter and interference. Larger diameter pins have a higher resistance to bending forces. This in turn can reduce the stresses at the bone–pin interface.[1] The limit to increasing pin size is set by the diameter of the bone in which the pin is inserted. A hole exceeding 20% of the diameter of the bone will reduce torsional strength by 34%, and if the hole size is greater than 50%, the reduction is 62%.[2] In practice, it is advisable to keep pin sizes to within a third of the diameter of the bone to reduce the risk of fracture on removal of the half pin. Interference is a measure of the grip the pin has of bone; traditionally it is at its maximum at the time of pin insertion and may decrease gradually as the fixator is loaded. Manufacturers have sought to maintain the grip on bone by altering the material properties or surface coatings of the pin. One technology that has shown promise in comparative studies and proven itself in clinical use is hydroxyapatite (HA) coating of the threaded portion of the pin. This causes bone hold to increase with time with increased extraction torques.

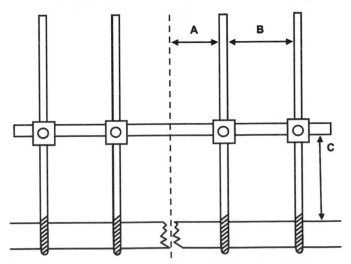

Fig. 1. Factors influencing stability of a simple monolateral external fixator. (A) Pin to fracture distance. (B) Pin to pin distance. (C) Bar to bone distance.

The mode of application and configuration of the fixator is important. Three pins in any one bone segment have increased stiffness and are advised for simple configuration constructs.[3] Avoiding thermal necrosis on insertion with cool irrigation is paramount (greater than 50°C can cause bone necrosis); the near/near, far/far principle of insertion produces biomechanically stable fixation and the stability is reduced as distance from pin to fracture increases.[4] The pins should be placed outside the zone of injury (including fracture hematoma) if at all possible and also be placed to allow access for further intervention (eg, plastic surgical reconstruction). The distance of the connecting bar from the bone is determined by the soft tissues, but stability is improved if the bar is as close to the bone, allowing of course for appropriate pin site care and the provision for swelling.

Although there are many circular and hybrid external fixators on the market that can be used for salvage of nonunion and malunion of the foot and ankle, the authors' experience is mainly with the systems described here.

The Ilizarov Method

In 1949, Gavril Ilizarov moved to Kurgan, Western Siberian Russia, where he perfected his technique treating war wounded with limb-threatening injuries using rings and tensioned fine wires connected by threaded bars. The basis of the method is that the bone is subjected to continual external tension.[5] By altering the direction and speed of loading, deformities may be corrected, and bone may be lengthened by distraction osteogenesis. This has been developed into the modern-day Ilizarov method. Fixation to supporting rings is achieved with 1.5 mm and 1.8 mm smooth or olive wires. Changing from a 1.5 mm to a 1.8 mm wire can increase stiffness parameters by 20%.[6] Inserting wires at least 50° to each other, with two or more wires per ring of correct diameter and chosen material (carbon fiber is less rigid in all parameters) can increase stability and minimize angulation and rotation. With appropriate load transfer and beam loading of wires, one practically ca eliminate any bending moments. The Ilizarov (Smith and Nephew, Memphis, Tennessee) generally relies on staged treatment for complex deformities using hinges and translation prespecified by the surgeon for each individual case to achieve correction.

The marriage of half pin fixators and ring constructs introduced hybrid frames to trauma and reconstruction surgery. The Taylor spatial frame (TSF, Smith and Nephew), a recent addition to the external fixation armamentarium, is an alternative to the Ilizarov method for stabilizing and treating peri-articular fractures or complex deformity.

The Taylor Spatial Frame

The Taylor spatial frame was introduced to global orthopedics in the mid-1990s.[7] It is a design based on the Stewart platform model, which has been adapted in numerous fields including flight simulation, crane technology, and satellite positioning systems.[8] Its use in orthopedics has helped develop an effective tool for multiplanar deformity correction and increasingly now in fracture management. It has a range of ring sizes that are only available in aluminum alloy, and therefore radio-opaque, which are connected by telescopic struts. Fixation to bone is achieved by either fine wires (diameters 1.6 mm/1.8 mm) or half pins (hybrid fixation). The main advantage of the TSF is the ability to correct angular, rotational, and translational deformity simultaneously around each of their three axes, a so-called six-axis correction. This is achieved through its six-strut design; the six struts are all independently adjustable to reorientate the rings relative to one another and ultimately achieve correction with 6° of freedom through one frame. Internet-based software generated with the TSF can plan the correction required to aid frame application, and the patient can follow a prescription of regular frame adjustments to correct the deformity. The TSF plan can be used for either single-stage correction of a complex deformity or the staged correction of a deformity. The TSF software now contains specialist tools for correcting foot and ankle deformity.

In surgery of the foot and ankle, both the Ilizarov method and the TSF are excellent treatment choices for t stabilizing complex peri-articular fractures. More frequently, however, they are used for correcting foot and ankle deformity. The Ilizarov has been used for over 50 years, however the TSF is a relative newcomer with less than 20 years in practice. Both methods are valid techniques and appropriate for treating what can be very challenging deformities. Both require meticulous preoperative planning for the relevant osteotomies and accurate placement of wires and rings. Use of the Ilizarov technique certainly depends more upon the surgeon to calculate the axis of the hinges and the rate of distraction; however, both techniques are liable to failure if sound principles are not followed.

Whichever method is used in fracture stabilization or correcting foot and ankle deformity, certain guidelines should be followed:

The construct should be stable.
The bone fixation should be stable.
The soft tissues and neurovascular structures should be treated with due care and
    attention.

TREATMENT OF SIMPLE ANKLE FRACTURES BY EXTERNAL FIXATION

Simple ankle fractures are a common presentation in emergency departments and orthopedic units. Most unstable pattern injuries are treated with initial plaster cast immobilization followed by internal fixation. Cross-ankle external fixation using half pins and bars, however, can be helpful in acute stabilization of these fractures in several clinical scenarios. First, the inherent stability of the fracture may be so poor (ie, trimalleolar with large posterior fragment) that maintained reduction may not be possible with temporary cast immobilization while the swelling settles; a secondary advantage is that it allows the surgeon to assess the degree of swelling without risking destabilization of the fracture by repeatedly opening the plaster splint. This approach also may be useful in open fractures where skin grafting may be necessary, so as to allow change of dressings and prevent tissue maceration.

As explained, there are significant advantages of temporary external fixation of displaced ankle fractures before definitive management, but a poorly applied spanning external fixator has more disadvantages than benefits. Meticulous attention to technique is essential in preventing complications, and the fixator configuration must be designed for maximum bony and soft tissue stability (**Fig. 2**).

Fixator Configurations for Spanning External Fixation of Ankle

Proximal fixation
Half-pins (5 mm or 6 mm) are used in the tibia. A biplanar configuration of the pins (one pin passed anteroposterior and one anteromedial to posterolateral) and spread of fixation in the tibia assure the best mechanical advantage.

Distal fixation
A transfixing 5 mm pin in the os calcis provides good stability. Care must be taken to avoid neurovascular injury. An area posterior to the midpoint of the line joining the posteroinferior point of the medial os calcis and the tip of the medial malleolus and an area posterior to the one-third mark of a line joining the navicular tuberosity to

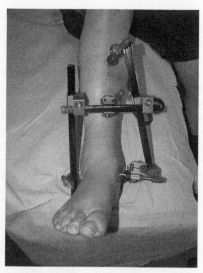

Fig. 2. An ankle-spanning external fixator.

the posteroinferior point of the os calcis provide safe zones,[9] although the medial calcaneal nerve is always at risk.

A mediolateral pin in the neck of the talus provides excellent near control for an ankle fracture, but can sometimes be difficult to insert; additionally, it is close to the distal extension of an anteromedial approach to the ankle.

A popular site for pin placement is to use a 4 mm or 5 mm pin in the base of the first metatarsal, crossing the first intermetatarsal space and gripping the base of the second metatarsal. The deep plantar branch of the dorsalis pedis artery, however, is consistently at risk with such pin placement,[10] and placement of the pin into the first metatarsal alone is safer.

External fixation also could be used in cases where the stability of the fracture is questionable or in the presence of poor skin quality often seen in diabetic patients, where infection would be a concern if open reduction and internal fixation were used. In these cases, if necessary, external fixation can be supplemented by percutaneous internal fixation with intramedullary fibular fixation or medial malleolar screws.

Open reduction internal fixation of ankle fractures is a common procedure undertaken in any orthopedic trauma unit. Complications may include nerve damage, swelling, stiffness, residual pain, and post-traumatic osteoarthritis. The procedure also may be complicated by malunion, nonunion, and infection.

Most malunions and nonunions are treated by removal of metalwork, freshening of the fracture site (with or without bone graft/biologic substitute, depending on whether it is atrophic), and repeat internal fixation. There are certain patient factors that may make this standard treatment of noninfective nonunions inappropriate. The most common of these is the neuropathic diabetic. There is frequently paucity of bone quality; however, this may be addressed by increasing the mechanical strength of the internal construct (eg, locking plates) and increasing the length of time non-weight-bearing and total length of time immobilized. Unfortunately, the patient mobilizing upon the fracture before it has united, either of his or her own volition or because of poor medical advice, can complicate the noninfective nonunion. In these cases, lack of protective pain sensation can allow complete destruction of the internal fixation and the bone to which it was applied. Reconstruction is not a feasible option with this presentation, and ankle (or even tibio-talo-calcaneal) arthrodesis should be undertaken. This may be achieved by standard internal fixation techniques. The soft tissues are often of dubious quality, however, and patients may have difficulty in following standard nonweight-bearing postoperative protocols. The authors therefore have a very low threshold for using a circular external fixator for the arthrodesis. This normally would be performed by means of a transfibular approach using an oscillating saw to obtain planar cuts (**Fig. 3**).

Large amounts of compression may be achieved by means of a highly stable construct that will allow immediate weight-bearing as tolerated mobilization. The frame normally is required for 12 to 18 weeks. To prevent this complication of the index internal fixation, the authors standard practice is to keep patients nonweight-bearing for at least 8 weeks, with total immobilization being at least 3 months.

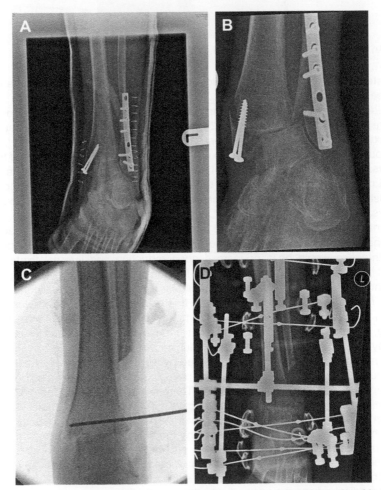

Fig. 3. A diabetic, neuropathic ankle fracture revised to ankle arthrodesis. (*A*) Ankle internal fixation. (*B*) Failure of internal fixation. (*C*) Transfibular ankle arthrodesis. (*D*) Ilizarov stabilization of arthrodesis.

PILON FRACTURES

Pilon fractures constitute a vast spectrum of distal tibial fractures, ranging from the partial articular fractures, to the complex, high-energy total articular fractures with metaphyseo–diaphyseal dissociation (MDD). The goal of treatment of such fractures is to restore the articular surface and restore the MDD.

Partial Articular Fractures

The simplest partial articular fractures lend themselves to closed reduction and internal fixation with screws, but most such fractures are treated by open reduction, interfragmentary screw fixation of the articular surface, and a neutralization plate. The planning of the operative approach depends on the specific subtype of fracture,[11] as the fracture line in such fractures can be quite variable. Problems such as wound breakdown complicated internal fixation in the past. A careful analysis of the axial CT scans to plan the surgical approach, an appropriate period of waiting to allow the soft tissue swelling to settle, and minimizing stripping of soft tissues during surgery have resulted in a large reduction in complication rates. Newer low-profile plates, particularly those with multiangular locking options for the metaphyseal bone, have reduced this problem further.

Total Articular Fractures

In addition to restoration of the articular surface, the MDD needs to be restored in these injuries. There is no argument that restoration of the articular surface necessitates an open reduction, with incisions based on the direction of the fracture lines on the axial CT scan. This approach may be anterolateral, posterolateral, or medial, depending on fracture configuration.

Restoration of the MDD can be performed either with plate fixation or with an external fixator. Plate fixation was popularized in the 1960s and 1970s, but increasing complications with its use in high-energy fractures[12,13] saw a trend toward external fixation for these fractures.[14] A randomized controlled trial of internal versus external fixation for such fractures was abandoned because of a high incidence of complications with internal fixation.[15] Although the trial itself was subject to criticism because of the selection of timing of operative intervention, the results did focus attention on catastrophic problems with fixation of such fractures.

Internal fixation after a period of spanning monolateral fixation has been reported to show a significant decrease in complications,[16,17] and there is published literature suggesting that internal fixation provides better outcomes than external fixation in such fractures.[18]

Critics of internal fixation, however, state that a subanalysis of these studies will reveal a high incidence of complications with internal fixation of high-energy fractures, including open fractures.

The use of monolateral fixators in the definitive treatment of these fractures has been described.[19] A circular frame, however, has many distinct advantages:

The use of fine wires allows fixation in the often small metaphyseal piece of bone
The mechanics of the circular fixator allow beam loading and axial micromotion and eliminate shear, all of which are especially conducive to fracture healing in these difficult scenarios.
The use of a circular frame permits the surgeon to fine-tune alignment of the fracture during the healing process. Such fine-tuning may be necessary in comminuted fractures, where the intraoperative image intensifier films do not

sometimes reveal malalignment of the MDD, and in cases with significant fragmentation, where a collapse during healing may lead to deformity.

The authors' preference is minimal periarticular internal fixation supplemented by an all-wire Ilizarov frame with four rods between the rings across the fracture where there is confidence perioperatively that alignment of the MDD is satisfactory. A technical review by Hutson covers the intraoperative steps in detail for treating acute pilon fractures.[20]

If there is doubt about alignment of the MDD, a TSF is used. If a decision to use a TSF is made, particular note must be made of the potential for decreased crossing angles with the TSF ring,[21] and the authors have a low threshold for supplementing distal fixation with a heel ring and crossing wires in the os calcis.

The personal practice adopted by the authors probably best reflects the views expressed by Watson and colleagues in 2000.[22] No one treatment will provide the best answer to the spectrum of injuries with which a pilon fracture presents. In cases with minimal soft tissue injury, internal fixation of the MDD after a period of spanning monolateral fixation is offered. In high-energy pilon fractures with gross fragmentation of the MDD, and those with severe open injuries, a circular frame to restore the continuity of the MDD is offered.

Malunion and nonunion are recognized complications of pilon fractures. These can be complicated by the state of the soft tissues, and by plastic reconstructive procedures, particularly in high-energy total articular fractures. The most common positions of malunions are varus, recurvatum, or a combination. Varus malunions commonly are found where the fibula has been plated laterally out to length. If the tibia is slow to unite, and the ankle syndesmosis is intact, then varus collapse will ensue. This may be treated by acute correction with a dome osteotomy of the tibia and fibula. This may be stabilized by internal fixation or with a circular external fixator. Two potential benefits of the latter are that more immediate weight-bearing may be undertaken, and fine tuning of the position can be achieved by gradual correction. Acute corrections, by opening or closing wedge osteotomy, are also popular techniques. They do not form part of the authors' standard practice because of the risks of delayed union/nonunion across the graft site with opening wedges and the additional leg length lost with a closing wedge. If there was additional loss of leg length because of an acute shortening being performed at the time of index reconstruction, then thought should be given to distraction osteogenesis. The same operative techniques can be utilized for treating recurvatum or combination deformities.

The key to treatment of nonunions is debridement. Obviously necrotic bone at the initial fracture site has no chance of healing, and a thorough debridement back to bleeding cancellous bone is necessary. It is also prudent to have a high index of suspicion that any cortical fragments left also may not be viable. The major treatment decision, after debridement, is whether reconstruction is possible, or if arthrodesis is necessary. For reconstruction to be possible, there needs to be approximately 2 cm of intact plafond metaphysis. Authors have described internal and external fixation techniques for performing this reconstruction. Internal fixation techniques using a blade plate have reported successful union rates of 75% to 100%.[23–25] There is interest as to whether lower-profile locking plates will have any additional benefit. Hypertrophic nonunions are a subgroup of nonunion patients highly amenable to external fixation. This is based upon the Ilizarov principle that hypertrophic nonunions may be treated with distraction and angular correction.[26] The authors' preference is to treat the reconstructable nonunions with internal fixation. If, however, there are poor soft tissues, severe bone loss, marked deformity, or infection present, then a circular external fixator is used.

If less than 2 cm of plafond metaphysis remains present, then an arthrodesis should be performed. The options for stabilization in arthrodesis are the same as those for reconstruction. Although it is possible to use standard methods of ankle arthrodesis fixation (eg, three cancellous screws), it is rare that the bone stock is of sufficient quality. A blade plate or locking plate therefore generally is used by means of a posterolateral approach. If the soft tissues anteriorly are of poor quality, then the posterior approach may be used successfully.[27] If extensive debridement has been performed, either at initial or secondary reconstruction, then distraction osteogenesis may be undertaken with intercalary transport. This can avoid the problems of wound closure with acute shortening. It is hoped that this will normalize gait by correcting the leg length discrepancy.

ANKLE AND PILON FIXATION INFECTIONS

Infection after internal fixation of ankle fractures can vary from being minor and superficial, resolving with appropriate oral antibiotic therapy, to deep infection resulting in wound breakdown and deep sepsis. Early deep wound infection is managed better aggressively. This consists of reopening the entire wound and debridement of all infected tissue including removal of loose and nonviable pieces of bone. An algorithm for treating infected ankle fixations is presented (**Fig. 4**).

An argument can be made for retaining internal fixation provided it is stable. On the contrary, it is the opinion of some surgeons, including the authors, that any potential biofilm never can be eradicated unless all metalwork is removed. A recent review suggests that 68% of infected cases where the metalwork was retained in the presence of infection went on to uncomplicated union, and 32% needed metalwork removal for union to take place.[28]

The authors believe in removal of all metalwork from the bone, and debridement of the screw holes and the surface of the fibula. Multiple samples (a minimum of three) are obtained from the soft tissues and the bone, and systemic antibiotic therapy is instituted only after samples are obtained.[29] Simpson and colleagues reported on effects of margin of clearance of the debridement.[30] Intralesional debridement was statistically significantly the worst, with all patients having recurrences of infection. There were no recurrences in patients who had a margin of excision greater than 5 mm. The rate of recurrence was 28% in patients who had a marginal excision (ie, less than 5 mm). All recurrences, however, were in type B hosts, those who had a predilection to infection or poor wound healing, as described by Cierney and Mader.[31] A standard technique to enable local administration of antibiotics is implantation of antibiotic-impregnated cement (PMMA) beads. If it is to be some time before the secondary procedure, the authors commonly use antibiotic-impregnated calcium sulfate. Mckee and colleagues reported its successful use, with a cure rate in 92% of 25 patients who had had postoperative osteomyelitis for a mean of 43 months before treatment.[32]

Soft tissue management is crucial for successful eradication of osteomyelitis. The wound should be closed following adequate debridement. If a soft-tissue defect is anticipated, consultation with a plastic surgeon must be done preoperatively, and a local flap or free flap should be performed after debridement. If wound closure cannot be performed, negative suction using a vacuum assisted closure (VAC) device can help healing. If facilities for this do not exist, a bead pouch[33] can be used as a temporizing measure, akin to treating open fractures, while awaiting plastic surgical cover.

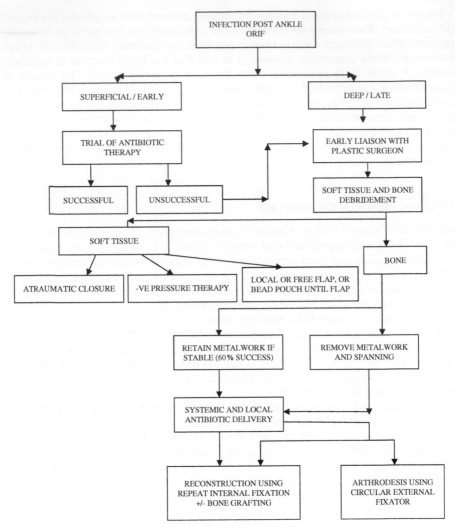

Fig. 4. An algorithm for the treatment of infected ankle fixations.

Skeletal stability is obtained using monolateral external fixation, with pins in the tibia, os calcis, and first metatarsal. Particular care must be taken when placing the tibial pins so as not to endanger the performance of a local fasciocutaneous flap; anteroposterior pin placement provides the safest corridor.

Systemic antibiotic therapy is instituted, initially on a best-guess protocol, after discussion with medical microbiology. Antibiotic therapy later is modified based on culture and sensitivity results, and 6 to 8 weeks of antibiotic therapy are recommended. Antibiotic levels may need monitoring, and the control of infection is gauged by serial estimations of inflammatory markers.

Reconstruction of the bone is performed after 4 to 6 weeks depending on the response to antibiotic therapy and debridement. Internal fixation can be redone, and special care must be taken to restore the length of the fibula, particularly if bony debridement has resulted in a defect; the length of the fibula can be estimated using the talocrural angle on the opposite side and reconstituting the same angle on the affected ankle. The plate can be fixed to the distal fragment, and the distal fragment jacked out using a laminar spreader. The plate then is fixed to the proximal fragment once the length of the fibula is re-established (**Fig. 5**).

The gap in the fibula is filled, either with autologous cancellous bone graft, which remains the gold standard, or a mixture of allograft and osteo-inductive agents that reduce the potential morbidity of bone graft harvest.

In cases of florid or long-standing infection after internal fixation of an ankle fracture, the infection can spread to the tibiotalar joint; this usually will be evident radiologically as bony destruction in this area. Such cases benefit from resection of the distal fibula and an arthrodesis of the ankle (**Fig. 6**). This is also true for treating infected pilon fractures (**Fig. 7**).

The main difference in the treatment of these fractures is the amount of resection that is usually necessary because of the extent of infection and necrotic bone. Although this is an on-table judgment, preoperative CT and MRI scans (with contrast) will give some indication to the extent of resection necessary. An arthrodesis in the presence of infection is performed best in two stages, as with reconstructive procedures, with local and systemic antibiotic therapy between the first and second stages.

Although such an arthrodesis can be performed using internal fixation,[27] it is the authors' personal preference to use fine wire circular fixation in such cases. At second look, debridement again is taken back to bleeding cancellous bone. Planar cuts then can be made. This generally is done having passed reference wires under image intensifier control so that the cuts are parallel to each other and perpendicular to the mechanical axis. Acute shortening then is performed if possible. The standard construct is to have a foot ring/plate with talar and calcaneal wires and two tibial rings approximately 15 cm above the ankle separated by 4 cm or 5 cm. Leg lengthening also may be performed by a proximal tibial corticotomy with an additional construct. If an acute shortening is not possible, or desirable, then intercalary transport may be performed. This will require a secondary procedure to prepare the arthrodesis site once docking has been performed.

MALUNION OF ANKLE ARTHRODESES AND TIBIAL MALUNIONS

Arthrodesis of the ankle requires meticulous preoperative planning to achieve fusion and to prevent deformity.[34] Malunited ankle arthrodeses can cause significant

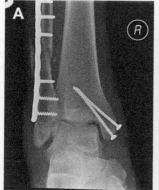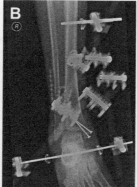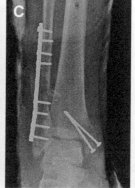

Fig. 5. Revision internal fixation for an infected ankle fracture fixation. (*A*) Ankle internal fixation. (*B*) Antibiotic beads with stabilizing, spanning external fixation. (*C*) Revision lateral plate fixation.

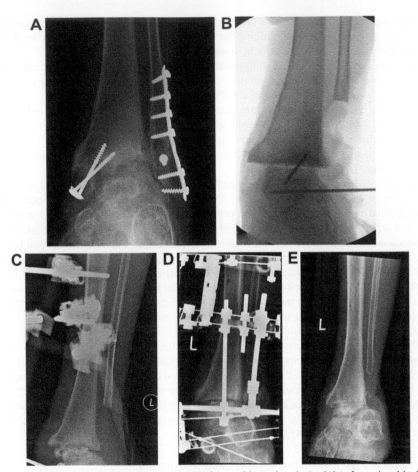

Fig. 6. Infected ankle fracture fixation revised to ankle arthrodesis. (*A*) Infected ankle fixation with significant articular destruction. (*B*) Obtaining planar cuts for arthrodesis at initial debridement. (*C*) Temporary spanning external fixation. (*D*) Ilizarov stabilization for arthrodesis. (*E*) Ankle arthrodesis.

problems with ambulation, and planning for surgical correction of these deformities is challenging.

Weight-bearing radiographs are important to calculate deformity. On the anteroposterior (AP) radiograph, a line passing midway through the width of the talus represents the middle on the frontal plane. On the assumption that there is no deformity in the foot, a line perpendicular to the weight-bearing foot on the lateral view, passing through the shadow of the lateral process of the talus, best represents the middle in the sagittal plane.[35] Mid-diaphyseal lines drawn through the tibia on both views represent the tibial axes. The point of intersection of the axes of the tibia and the foot will reveal the center of rotation of angulation (CORA).

Corrective osteotomies for malunited ankle fusions using the principles of gradual deformity correction using circular external fixation provide gratifying results.[36,37] The specific advantage of an adjustable circular frame in the correction of such deformity is that the position of the foot can be adjusted almost infinitesimally until a perfect position is achieved. Other advantages include maintenance of length and the decrease in the risk of neurologic abnormalities consequent on acute correction.

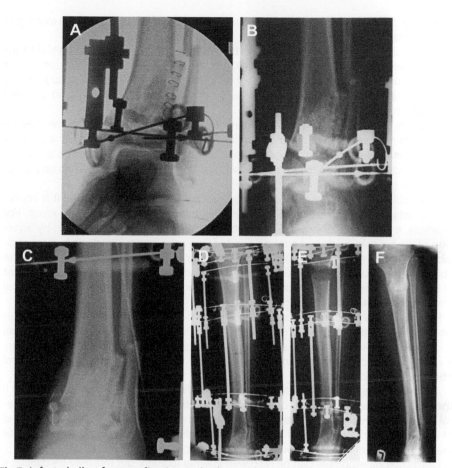

Fig. 7. Infected pilon fracture fixation revised to ankle arthrodesis. (*A*) Pilon fracture treated with an Ilizarov frame. (*B*) Loss of position with articular destruction. (*C*) Debridement with antibiotic beads and Ilizarov stabilization. (*D*) Simultaneous lengthening with ankle arthrodesis for significant bone loss. (*E*) Proximal corticotomy for distraction osteogenesis. (*F*) Healed corticotomy and ankle arthrodesis.

Such osteotomies, particularly those for recently malunited fusions, are performed best at a supramalleolar level (ie, the osteotomy is performed at a site away from the true CORA).[38] Thus, the bone ends will need to be translated to achieve correction of the mechanical axis. Such translation will have to be accurately monitored radiologically and clinically to achieve ideal correction.

A malunited tibial fracture can cause asymmetrical loading of adjacent joints, and has its most pronounced effect on the joint closest to it (ie, proximal tibial malunions tend to alter the mechanical axis of the limb to a greater degree and cause abnormal loading of either the lateral or medial compartment of knee), and distal tibial malunions produce alteration of the axis of the tibiotalar joint.

Experimental studies in cadavers[39] showed that angular deformity in the lower tibia altered tibiotalar mechanics significantly. Interestingly, these studies showed that malunion in the sagittal plane (procurvatum and recurvatum) produced more changes in the contact area of the tibiotalar joint than malunion in the coronal plane. In addition to angular deformities, translational malunion also can cause asymmetrical loading of the tibiotalar joint.

Tibial malunions causing symptoms in the ankle usually result from distal tibial fractures. Deformity may be obvious clinically, and the condition of the soft tissues around the malunion must be assessed. The degree of free movement in the subtalar joint and any deformity in the foot must be checked, as this may have a role to play in planning deformity correction.

A mobile subtalar joint can compensate for deformity in the ankle in the coronal plane. The normal range of about 30° of inversion and 15° of eversion in the subtalar joint means that up to about 30° of valgus orientation in the ankle and up to about 15° of varus still can be compensated in the subtalar area, and the heel still can be placed flat on the ground.

An established compensatory deformity may lead to a contracture, and it is important to establish the presence of such contractures before deformity correction. For example, a valgus malunion of a distal tibial fracture may be compensated by inversion of the subtalar joint, and over a period of time may lead to fixed varus in the subtalar joint. If this contracture is not appreciated, and if correction of the valgus in the tibia is performed, the heel will end up in decompensated varus. Therefore, movement of the subtalar joint in the direction of the correction is a prerequisite before surgical correction of distal tibial deformity.

Radiological analysis is performed using weight-bearing films. The CORA is calculated using the intersection of the proximal tibial mechanical axis (mid-diaphyseal line) and the distal tibial mechanical axis. If the distal fragment is small, the mid-diaphyseal line may be difficult to draw, and the mechanical axis is drawn using a lateral distal tibial angle of 89°.[40]

A corrective osteotomy ideally is performed at the CORA, but this may be difficult if the CORA is close to the joint, or if poor regeneration is anticipated because of sclerotic bone around the site of the malunion. In such cases, the osteotomy is performed at a site away from the level of the CORA, but deliberate translation may need to be performed to normalize the mechanical axis, using Osteotomy Rule 2.[38]

Corrective osteotomies can be held with internal fixation, but this may be difficult if the planned correction is large, and if the soft tissues are not pliable or are scarred. Furthermore, combined translation–angulation deformities are simpler to correct gradually using the principles of distraction osteogenesis and employing a circular external fixator. Length of the affected bone also is restored best using an open-wedge osteotomy and gradual correction.

Depending on the surgeon's choice, an Ilizarov frame or a TSF can be used for deformity correction. The authors' personal preference is to use an Ilizarov frame with hinges and motors for simple angular deformities, and a TSF for combined translation–angulation deformities or where the osteotomy is away from the CORA, thus needing secondary translation (**Fig. 8**).

A stable frame is applied, using reference wires or half-pins perpendicular to the long axis of the bone. Rings then are built on to this, resulting in a frame construct mimicking the deformity.

A low-energy division of the bone is performed using the technique in which the surgeon is most experienced, and considering soft-tissue scarring. Such osteotomies may be performed with osteotomes alone, multiple drill holes connected with an osteotome, or with a Gigli saw.[41] The authors' personal preference is to use the drill and osteotome technique. The fixator is assembled around the osteotomy, either using the six-strut configuration of the TSF or the hinges and motors of a traditional Ilizarov frame.

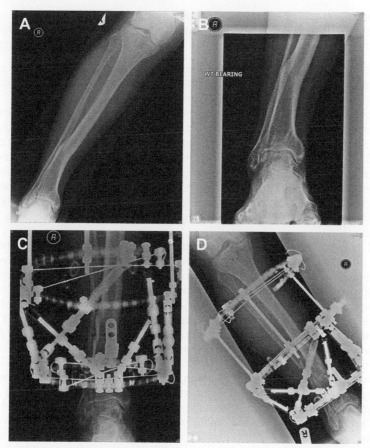

Fig. 8. Correction of a tibial malunion with medial ankle arthritis. (*A*) AP radiograph of tibia and fibula demonstrating malunion. (*B*) AP radiograph of ankle demonstrating medial ankle arthritis. (*C*) AP radiograph 2 days after osteotomy and application of the Taylor spatial frame. (*D*) AP radiograph after correction.

The structure at risk is assessed (usually the bone at the base of the opening wedge). A maximum distraction of 1 mm/d at this area is built into the planning protocol, and gradual correction of the osteotomy is started about 7 days after surgery. A stable frame allows weight-bearing as tolerated, and serial radiographs are obtained to ensure full correction of the mechanical axis.

The frame is removed once the newly formed regenerate is consolidated; this consolidation is evidenced radiologically by the formation of at least three cortices on two orthogonal views, and clinically by comfortable weight-bearing with gradual disassembly of the external fixator.

The Equinus Ankle Deformity

Any post-traumatic foot and ankle deformity presents a significant challenge to the orthopedic surgeon. The acquired, soft tissue equinus deformity secondary to trauma can result from conditions such as:

Contractures from burn scars
Long-term immobilization

A complication of limb-lengthening procedures
Contractures following compartment syndromes, crush injuries, scar contractures, and neurologic damage

Equinus deformity induces a tip-toe gait pattern with complete loss of heel strike at initial contact. The incidence of this condition has increased over recent years, with increasing numbers of road traffic collisions and subsequent limb salvage.

Many patients, especially burn patients, will have poor tissue quality secondary to contractures; therefore surgeons may want to avoid more invasive, open techniques involving Achilles tendon lengthening and capsular releases, for risk of wound complications. Single-stage open correction also may be associated with higher rates of neurovascular injury, and prophylactic tarsal tunnel release has been recommended for correction greater than 10°.[42] Even in gradual corrections, tarsal tunnel syndrome or peroneal nerve lesions can occur and can be released surgically with continuation of frame treatment[43]; alternatively, they may resolve by simply slowing the rate of correction.

In mild post-traumatic equinus deformities of less than 20°, open correction may produce good results, but correction beyond this may require other interventions such as hind foot osteotomies or gradual fine wire correction. It must be remembered that a mild deformity of less than 20° may be simply amenable to serial stretches and physiotherapy. Moderate deformities of 20° to 40° may be correctable with soft tissue releases and immobilization, and severe equinus deformity (greater than 40°) usually cannot be corrected by simple open releases in isolation.[44] Combining open Achilles lengthening, scar excision, free tissue grafting, and Ilizarov correction may be required for significant contractures of more than 45° secondary to massive soft tissue injury.[45]

Gradual correction using an Ilizarov frame may involve constrained or unconstrained hinged frames. Constrained frames involve fixed rotating hinges, whereas unconstrained frames use the ankle joint as a natural hinge. Tsuchiya and colleagues described both techniques in series of 16 patients and found no difference in correction achieved (32.9° and 36.1° improvements of dorsiflexion, $P=.58$). Tsuchiya, however, stressed that the natural or unconstrained hinge system needs to be monitored carefully for problems such as talar subluxation.[46]

For treating an acquired equinus, recurrence of the deformity is one complication documented in the literature.[47,48] Authors argue whether the period of rigid immobilization postoperatively affects the rate of recurrence.[46,49,50] It is more likely that the etiology of the deformity (ie, burn deformities)[51] can have up to 75% recurrence—especially in children because of continual bony growth with tight contracted soft tissues—has more of an influence. Patient compliance with postoperative stretches and splints is a factor,[48] as is the time from injury to treatment.

When considering correction of an equinus deformity, the surgeon and the patient need to be very clear regarding the possible outcomes. Patients must be made aware that an improvement is likely; however, recurrence is a problem. In mild deformities, physical therapy is a valuable option. At the more severe end of the spectrum, as with any fine wire fixator intervention, patient compliance is paramount, so careful patient selection is vital.

CALCANEAL FRACTURES

Stephens and Sanders proposed a classification system for calcaneal malunions.[52] Type 1 malunions have a lateral wall exostosis without subtalar arthrosis or hind foot malalignment. Type 2 have a lateral wall exostosis and subtalar arthrosis with hind foot malalignment that is less than 10°. Type 3 malunions demonstrate the lateral exostosis and subtalar arthrosis, but with this subgroup, the hind foot deformity this exceeds 10°. Nonunion of calcaneal fractures is uncommon, with Zwipp and colleagues reporting a rate of 1.3%.[53]

Type 1 malunions result from intra-articular fractures of the calcaneus that may be treated with a lateral wall exostosectomy and surgical treatment of any effect on the peroneal tendons, which may have been abraded or subluxated by the exostosis.

Surgical treatment of type 2 malunions involves a lateral wall exostosectomy and subtalar arthrodesis. Whether this can be an in situ arthrodesis or requires a distraction bone block arthrodesis depends on the presence of collapse of the calcaneus.[54,55] This collapse will have the effect of producing a pes planus, with a rocker bottom deformity caused by superior translation of the calcaneal tuberosity and the collapse of the body and neck. The point of initial contact and stance therefore may be distal to the heel pad. The collapse also may have a secondary dorsiflexing effect on the talar head declination angle, thereby restricting ankle dorsiflexion because of impingement against the distal tibia.

Subtalar arthrodesis alone may be insufficient to correct the axial malalignment in the type 3 mal unions. This is because the deformity arises not just from any depression of the articular surface but from deformity within the body of the calcaneus itself. In this situation, a simple lateral translation or Dwyer closing wedge calcaneal osteotomy may be used for varus deformities, and a medial translation osteotomy for valgus deformities. This can be performed in addition to the subtalar arthrodesis.

The deformities also may be addressed with by using circular external fixators with or without distraction osteogenesis. There are three main scenarios when these are of benefit. First, a paucity of soft tissues may be present because of the index fracture being open or large amounts of soft tissue contusion (eg, high energy or blast injury), postoperative infection, or soft tissue contractures secondary to marked superior translation at the calcaneal tuberosity. Second, a stiff but nonpainful subtalar joint may be present obviating the need for an arthrodesis. Third, the complexity of the deformity may be challenging to correct acutely. This complexity may be enhanced by severe disuse osteoporosis that may make successful and stable internal fixation difficult.

In atypical type 1 malunions where there is a lateral wall exostosis, loss of the height of the calcaneus, but the subtalar joint does not need to be addressed (either because this is unaffected or stiffened and painless), distraction osteogenesis may be used to correct the calcaneal pitch.

A lateral approach is used for the exostosectomy, and through this approach, an oblique calcaneal osteotomy may be performed. Distraction then can be used to rotate the inferior pole of the calcaneal tuberosity in a caudal direction (**Fig. 9**). The same approach may be used in type 2 or type 3 malunions in conjunction with a triple arthrodesis if it is felt that the soft tissue environment would not allow for an acute distraction bone block arthrodesis.

Multiplanar deformities of the whole foot secondary to a neglected calcaneal malunion (with or without other hind foot or midfoot trauma) also may be addressed with gradual correction using a circular external fixator. These may be either type 2 or type 3 malunions. A V-osteotomy is a double-limbed osteotomy that can be used to correct nonmatching deformities of the forefoot and hind foot, around the body of the talus. The V is centered around the body of the talus and the thalamic portion of the calcaneus. The posterior limb extends from the calcaneal tuberosity through the inferior calcaneus, creating a posterior tuberosity segment. Anterior limb extends to the inferior calcaneus through the calcaneal and talar necks, creating

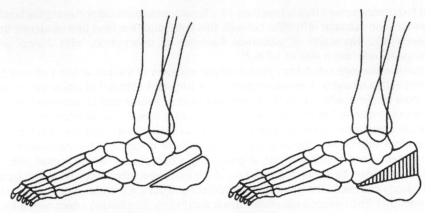

Fig. 9. Osteotomy for distraction osteogenesis of calcaneus.

an anterior forefoot segment (**Fig. 10**). A stiff subtalar joint is a prerequisite for this osteotomy. Separate posterior and forefoot rings therefore may be attached with the necessary separate dynamic connections being made, depending upon the type of circular external fixator used. Once the gradual correction has been performed and the regenerate is consolidating, it is possible to perform a secondary subtalar arthrodesis, which may be stabilized using the frame with or without supplementary internal fixation.

Calcaneal nonunion is an uncommon sequela of calcaneal fractures. Molloy and colleagues reported on a series of 15 fractures, of which four had concomitant osteomyelitis. These were treated with a bone block distraction arthrodesis and internal fixation. Fourteen patients (94%) went on to union, with an average of two reconstructive procedures. The eventual outcome was a subtalar arthrodesis in 10 (67%) cases and triple arthrodesis in 4 (27%). The one nonunion was of the patient's own volition, as he was asymptomatic after initial debridement for concomitant osteomyelitis, and he declined further surgery. There were, however, three wound dehiscences; all of these patients received a local rotational flap. These three patients had all had wound dehiscences from the index fracture fixation.[56] In this subgroup of patients, the

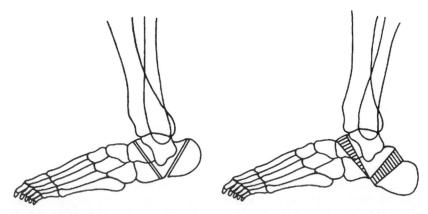

Fig. 10. A V osteotomy.

authors believe that it is prudent to discuss the risk of acute correction and to also offer treatment of the nonunion without full correction of the calcaneal tuberosity. The residual deformity then can be corrected with a secondary distraction osteogenesis of the tuberosity once union was achieved.

Another indication for circular external fixation and the salvage of nonunion calcaneal fractures is in the treatment of complex calcaneal fractures with bony defects from land mine blast injuries. Gür and colleagues reported on 21 patients who had large residual bony defects or massive calcaneal destruction following blast injuries.[57] Soft tissue injuries were classified according to the method of Oestern and Tscherne.[58] All patients had grade 3 soft tissue injuries. Soft tissue defects that could not be closed were treated with free flap coverage, followed by a slit skin graft. Before definitive surgery, the calcaneal bone loss ranged from 20% to 100%. The surgical technique used was, following thorough debridement, an oblique osteotomy of the calcaneus, talus, or posterior aspect of the distal tibia depending on the magnitude of the posterior hindfoot defect. This osteotomy then was rotated around the coronal plane to recreate a heel. The Ilizarov technique was used for the distraction osteogenesis. The frame was applied at an average of 10 months following index injury. The authors managed to achieve four excellent, 11 good, five fair, and two poor results in what were severe and complex injuries.

TALAR NECK AND MIDFOOT FRACTURES

Talar neck fractures are the most common fractures of the talus, accounting for over 50% of cases. The Hawkins classification,[59] modified by Canale and Kelly,[60] is based upon displacement of the fractures and any associated subluxation or dislocation (**Box 1**).

Canale and Kelly reported good-to-excellent outcomes in 59% of 71 patients at an average of 12.7 years.[60] The reasons for the less good outcomes were post-traumatic arthritis and avascular necrosis. The rates of avascular necrosis were 10% of type 1, 50% of type 2, 85% of type 3, and 100% of type 4. Vallier and colleagues reported rates of 54% of post-traumatic osteoarthritis and a rate of 49% of avascular necrosis.[61] Salvage of avascular necrosis of the talus can be a demanding procedure depending on the extent of the involvement of the talus and any associated deformity. MRI is crucial in preoperative planning to accurately delineate the margins of healthy bone stock. One should bear in mind, however, the resection limits may be larger than indicated on MRI if additional bone, although viable, is of poor quality. In using internal fixation, there are two alternatives for addressing the defect. An acute shortening may be performed, or the defect may be filled with bone graft (most likely allograft in view of the necessary volume), perhaps supplemented by biologic substitutes with or without an implantable electrical bone stimulator. It is, however, challenging to achieve union

---

Box 1
The Hawkins classification of talar neck fractures

Type 1—talar neck fracture, undisplaced

Type 2—talar neck fracture with associated sub-talar joint dissociation

Type 3—talar neck fracture with both ankle and subtalar joint dissociation

Type 4 (added by Canale and colleagues)—talar neck fracture with associated talo–navicular dissociation

across large defects of grafting because of the relatively hypovascular status of the talus. Achieving fixation also may be challenging, and acute shortening because of the small remnants of talus remaining. Intramedullary retrograde nails are among the standard methods of internal fixation of tibio-talo-calcaneal fusions. Young and colleagues[62] found that because of the fixed nature of the distal locking screw holes, these screws were placed in a suboptimal position. This positioning problem will be accentuated with the larger volumes of debridement that are necessary in the presence of avascular necrosis as compared with for more standard post-traumatic osteoarthritis. It also has been shown that the Ilizarov fixator provides a biomechanically stiffer construct than intramedullary devices.[63] Blade plates can be used for internal stabilization, either using a posterior or posterolateral approach, with excellent results.[64] There have been more recent biomechanical studies that suggest that locking plates provide greater mechanical stability and load to failure than blade plates.[65] These both, however, involve a relatively large amount of soft tissue stripping to allow plate placement and give the patient a leg length discrepancy if an acute shortening is performed. Circular external fixators are a rival alternative for stabilization. Because of the dynamic ability of these fixators, large amounts of compression may be achieved, as well as allowing secondary correction of any deformity. In addition, distraction osteogenesis may be performed using a proximal tibial osteotomy to correct leg length discrepancy, if this is thought to be of clinical significance. The frame configuration will be similar to that as outlined in the sections on salvage of pilon fractures and nonunion of ankle arthrodesis.

MIDFOOT MALUNIONS

Midtarsal and Lisfranc's injuries include a spectrum of disorders from sprains to severe disassociations of the midfoot with associated soft tissue injuries. This section will deal with sequelae at the more severe end of the spectrum. Up to 81% of these injuries are in multiply injured people.[66] This demonstrates the level of force involved in the injuries to overcome the strong bony and ligamentous support of these joints. A thorough anatomic classification scheme was reported by Myerson and colleagues,[66] which was based upon the segmental patterns of injury and the forces involved. Anatomically, however, it is often simpler to describe the injury in terms of the column of the foot that is affected (**Fig 11**).[67]

Myerson also has classified the mechanism of injury as being direct or indirect.[66] Direct injuries are caused by a direct crushing injury to the tarsometatarsal joints. These injuries frequently are comminuted and are complicated by soft tissue damage and a higher incidence of compartment syndrome. Because of the direct nature of the force of injury, the sagittal deformity tends to be plantarward. Indirect injuries usually occur with a plantarflexed foot with the metatarsals planted on the ground. The momentum of the body then produces a torque force with rotation, abduction, and dorsal tension. Although the force of injury is less, compartment syndrome still may ensue, and due diligence should be taken.

Treatment of these injuries has progressed over the past few decades from closed treatment, closed treatment stabilized with wires, to primary internal fixation with or without arthrodesis. Results have improved in this spectrum of disorders. Even in the presence of ideal anatomic fixation, however, results may be varied depending on the level of comminution and crushing from the index injury.

Malunions of these injuries usually involve an abducted forefoot and midfoot with a secondary forefoot driven calcaneovalgus. This abduction can be caused by malunion of the fractures, chronic subluxation of any affected joints, and failure to regain

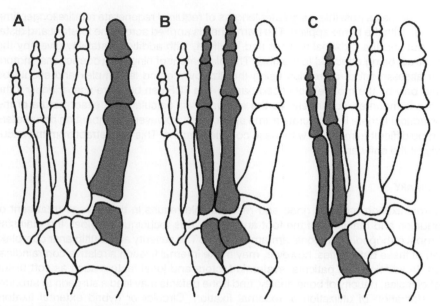

Fig. 11. Columnar classification of injury of the midfoot. (*A*) Medial. (*B*) Middle. (*C*) Lateral.

the length of the crushed lateral column at the initial reconstruction. In addition, there also may be deformity in the sagittal plane depending on whether the index mechanism of injury was direct (causing plantar displacement) or indirect (causing dorsal displacement).

Salvage of these deformities may be treated successfully by arthrodesis using acute correction and internal fixation. The level of difficulty of succeeding in this procedure, however, depends upon the complexity of this deformity. The most severe end of the spectrum involves deformity in the axial and sagittal planes together with a rotatory deformity. This can be corrected acutely by taking triplane wedges across the midfoot. The size of wedge may be determined preoperatively from weight-bearing anteroposterior and lateral radiographs. To help ensure this plan is followed intraoperatively, guidewires should be driven along the limbs of the proposed osteotomy, and the correct positioning can be checked fluoroscopically. The osteotomies then may be performed along these guidewires using an oscillating saw or osteotomes. Rotation then may be corrected manually before internally fixing with compression screws and plates. Especially in direct crush injuries, however, there may be concerns for the soft tissue envelope (and the amount of stripping necessary) and a degree of foreshortening that may occur with the excision of this wedge. In severe cases, this foreshortening may leave a cosmetic and functional shortening of the foot, as well as turning the longitudinal approaches into more oval wounds that can be difficult to close with nonpliable soft tissue. In these circumstances, circular external frames provide a viable option. If there is a correctable calcaneovalgus without arthritis of the subtalar joint, a medial translation calcaneal osteotomy may be performed in standard fashion and internally fixed. The forefoot and midfoot deformity then can be included in the dynamic part of the frame. Affected joints can be prepared with osteotomes by a combination of medial and lateral approaches. If an oscillating saw is to be used, then great care should be taken not to cause thermal necrosis, as this will affect the quality of the regeneration directly. The aim with this joint preparation is to remove as little bone as possible, as greater lengths of required regenerate require longer time periods with the frame applied. The frame then is applied across the forefoot and distal midfoot and the proximal midfoot and hindfoot, with additional stability given by the construct being attached to the tibia. The placement of hinges as correctional motors and assessment of correction using the Ilizarov method is complex and should be used only by the most experienced hands. The TSF can be more user-friendly if the frame is mounted accurately, as the software will calculate the exact nature of the correction. If there is inaccurate frame application, however, the mounting parameters can be difficult to measure with these complex frames. This will detract from the accuracy of the software.

SUMMARY

Internal fixation provides good and reproducible results in the salvage treatment of nonunion and malunion of the foot and ankle. This technique provides the mainstay of most orthopedic surgeons' armamentarium. The severity and multiplanar complexities of these deformities, however, may make internal fixation a relative contraindication. In addition, the patients' systemic factors and local factors such as soft tissue deficiencies, paucity of bone quality, and bone defects may lead a surgeon to stronger consideration of utilization of external fixation. Circular or hybrid external fixators certainly would be considered the method of choice in the presence of infection for the salvage of nonunion and malunion of foot and ankle trauma.

REFERENCES

1. Huiskes R, Chao EY, Crippen TE. Parametric analyses of pin–bone stresses in external fracture fixation devices. J Orthop Res 1985;3:341–9.
2. Edgerton BC, An KN, Morrey BF. Torsional strength reduction due to cortical defects in bone. J Orthop Res 1990;8:851–5.
3. Briggs BT, Chao EY. The mechanical performance of the standard Hoffmann-Vidal external fixation apparatus. J Bone Joint Surg Am 1982;64:566–73.
4. Huiskes R, Chao EY. Guidelines for external fixation frame rigidity and stresses. J Orthop Res 1986;4:68–75.
5. Kirienko A, Villa A, Calhoun J. Introduction. In: Ilizarov technique for complex foot and ankle deformities. New York: Marcel Dekker Ltd; 2004. p. 1–25.
6. Kummer FJ. Biomechanics of the Ilizarov external fixator. Clin Orthop Relat Res 1992;280:11–4.
7. Taylor JC. Complete characterisation of a 6-axes deformity; complete correction with a new external fixator "The spatial frame". Presented at the Annual Meeting of ASAMI North America. Atlanta, February 21, 1996.
8. Stewart D. Platform with six degrees of freedom. Proc Inst Mech Eng 1965;180: 371–86.
9. Casey D, McConnell T, Parekh S, et al. Percutaneous pin placement in the medial calcaneus: is anywhere safe? J Orthop Trauma 2002;16:26–9.
10. Barrett MO, Wade AM, Della Rocca GJ, et al. The safety of forefoot metatarsal pins in external fixation of the lower extremity. J Bone Joint Surg Am 2008;90: 560–4.
11. Topliss CJ, Jackson M, Atkins RM. Anatomy of pilon fractures of the distal tibia. J Bone Joint Surg Br 2005;87:692–7.
12. Kellam JF, Waddell JP. Fractures of the distal tibial metaphysis with intra-articular extension—the distal tibial explosion fracture. J Trauma 1979;19:593–601.

13. Dillin L, Slabaugh P. Delayed wound healing, infection, and nonunion following open reduction and internal fixation of tibial plafond fractures. J Trauma 1986; 26:1116–9.

14. McDonald MG, Burgess RC, Bolano LE, et al. Ilizarov treatment of pilon fractures. Clin Orthop Relat Res 1996;232–8.

15. Wyrsch B, McFerran MA, McAndrew M, et al. Operative treatment of fractures of the tibial plafond. A randomized, prospective study. J Bone Joint Surg Am 1996; 78:1646–57.

16. Sirkin M, Sanders R, DiPasquale T, et al. A staged protocol for soft tissue management in the treatment of complex pilon fractures. J Orthop Trauma 1999;13:78–84.

17. Blauth M, Bastian L, Krettek C, et al. Surgical options for the treatment of severe tibial pilon fractures: a study of three techniques. J Orthop Trauma 2001;15: 153–60.

18. Pollak AN, McCarthy ML, Bess RS, et al. Outcomes after treatment of high-energy tibial plafond fractures. J Bone Joint Surg Am 2003;85-A:1893–900.

19. Bonar SK, Marsh JL. Unilateral external fixation for severe pilon fractures. Foot Ankle 1993;14:57–64.

20. Hutson JJ. The treatment of distal tibia peri-articular fractures with circular ring fixators. In: Wiss D, editor. Master techniques in orthopaedic surgery–fractures. Philadelphia: Lippincott, Williams and Wilkins; 2006. p. 529–49.

21. Hawkins R, Calder P, Goodier D. Anatomical considerations and limitations of wire placement using the Taylor spatial frame. J Bone Joint Surg Br 2006;88-B: 170–1.

22. Watson JT, Moed BR, Karges DE, et al. Pilon fractures. Treatment protocol based on severity of soft tissue injury. Clin Orthop Relat Res 2000;375:78–90.

23. Chin KR, Nagarkatti DG, Miranda MA, et al. Salvage of distal tibia metaphyseal nonunions with the 90 degrees cannulated blade plate. Clin Orthop Relat Res 2003;409:241–9.

24. Reed LK, Mormino MA. Functional outcome after blade plate reconstruction of distal tibia metaphyseal nonunions: a study of 11 cases. J Orthop Trauma 2004;18:81–6.

25. Harvey EJ, Henley MB, Swiontkowski MF, et al. The use of a locking custom contoured blade plate for peri-articular nonunions. Injury 2003;34:111–6.

26. Hutson JJ. Salvage of pilon fracture nonunion and infection with circular tensioned wire fixation. Foot Ankle Clin 2008;13:29–68.

27. Sanders R, Pappas J, Mast J, et al. The salvage of open grade IIIB ankle and talus fractures. J Orthop Trauma 1992;6:201–8.

28. Rightmire E, Zurakowski D, Vrahas M. Acute infections after fracture repair: management with hardware in place. Clin Orthop Relat Res 2008;466:466–72.

29. Trampuz A, Zimmerli W. Diagnosis and treatment of infections associated with fracture-fixation devices. Injury 2006;37(Suppl 2):S59–66.

30. Simpson AH, Deakin M, Latham JM. Chronic osteomyelitis. The effect of the extent of surgical resection on infection-free survival. J Bone Joint Surg Br 2001;83:403–7.

31. Cierny G, Mader JT. Approach to adult osteomyelitis. Orthop Rev 1987;16: 259–70.

32. McKee MD, Wild LM, Schemitsch EH, et al. The use of an antibiotic-impregnated, osteoconductive, bioabsorbable bone substitute in the treatment of infected long bone defects: early results of a prospective trial. J Orthop Trauma 2002;16:622–7.

33. Keating JF, Blachut PA, O'Brien PJ, et al. Reamed nailing of open tibial fractures: does the antibiotic bead pouch reduce the deep infection rate? J Orthop Trauma 1996;10:298–303.

34. Ahmad J, Raikin SM. Ankle arthrodesis: the simple and the complex. Foot Ankle Clin 2008;13:381–400, viii.

35. Paley D, Herzenberg JE. Ankle and foot considerations. In: Paley D, Herzenberg JE, editors. Principles of deformity correction. Berlin: Springer; 2002. p. 571–645.

36. Katsenis D, Bhave A, Paley D, et al. Treatment of malunion and nonunion at the site of an ankle fusion with the Ilizarov apparatus. J Bone Joint Surg Am 2005; 87:302–9.

37. Paley D, Lamm BM, Katsenis D, et al. Treatment of malunion and nonunion at the site of an ankle fusion with the Ilizarov apparatus. Surgical technique. J Bone Joint Surg Am 2006;88(Suppl 1):119–34.

38. Paley D, Herzenberg JE. Osteotomy concepts and frontal plane realignment. In: Paley D, Herzenberg JE, editors. Principles of deformity correction. Berlin: Spinger; 2002. p. 99–154.

39. Tarr RR, Resnick CT, Wagner KS, et al. Changes in tibiotalar joint contact areas following experimentally induced tibial angular deformities. Clin Orthop Relat Res 1985;199:72–80.

40. Paley D, Herzenberg JE. Normal lower limb alignment and joint orientation. In: Paley D, Herzenberg JE, editors. Principles of deformity correction. Berlin: Springer; 2002. p. 1–18.

41. Paley D, Herzenberg JE. Hardware and Osteotomy considerations. In: Paley D, Herzenberg JE, editors. Principles of deformity correction. Berlin: Springer; 2002. p. 291–410.

42. Lamm BM, Paley D, Testani M, et al. Tarsal tunnel decompression in leg lengthening and deformity correction of the foot and ankle. J Foot Ankle Surg 2007;46:201–6.

43. Nogueira MP, Paley D, Bhave A, et al. Nerve lesions associated with limb-lengthening. J Bone Joint Surg Am 2003;85-A:1502–10.

44. Calhoun JH, Evans EB, Herndon DN. Techniques for the management of burn contractures with the Ilizarov fixator. Clin Orthop Relat Res 1992;280:117–24.

45. Hahn SB, Park HJ, Park HW, et al. Treatment of severe equinus deformity associated with extensive scarring of the leg. Clin Orthop Relat Res 2001; 393:250–7.

46. Tsuchiya H, Sakurakichi K, Uehara K, et al. Gradual closed correction of equinus contracture using the Ilizarov apparatus. J Orthop Sci 2003;8:802–6.

47. Huang SC. Soft tissue contractures of the knee or ankle treated by the Ilizarov technique. High recurrence rate in 26 patients followed for 3–6 years. Acta Orthop Scand 1996;67:443–9.

48. Emara KM, Allam MF, Elsayed MN, et al. Recurrence after correction of acquired ankle equinus deformity in children using Ilizarov technique. Strategies Trauma Limb Reconstr 2008;3:105–8.

49. Mendicino RW, Murphy LJ, Maskill MP, et al. Application of a constrained external fixator frame for treatment of a fixed equinus contracture. J Foot Ankle Surg 2008; 47:468–75.

50. Melvin JS, Dahners LE. A technique for correction of equinus contracture using a wire fixator and elastic tension. J Orthop Trauma 2006;20:138–42.

51. Carmichael KD, Maxwell SC, Calhoun JH. Recurrence rates of burn contracture ankle equinus and other foot deformities in children treated with Ilizarov fixation. J Pediatr Orthop 2005;25:523–8.

52. Stephens HM, Sanders R. Calcaneal malunions: results of a prognostic computed tomography classification system. Foot Ankle Int 1996;17:395–401.
53. Zwipp H, Tscherne H, Thermann H, et al. Osteosynthesis of displaced intraarticular fractures of the calcaneus. Results in 123 cases. Clin Orthop Relat Res 1993; 290:76–86.
54. Savva N, Saxby TS. In situ arthrodesis with lateral wall ostectomy for the sequelae of fracture of the os calcis. J Bone Joint Surg Br 2007;89:919–24.
55. Clare MP, Lee WE, Sanders RW. Intermediate to long-term results of a treatment protocol for calcaneal fracture malunions. J Bone Joint Surg Am 2005;87:963–73.
56. Molloy AP, Myerson MS, Yoon P. Symptomatic nonunion after fracture of the calcaneum. Demographics and treatment. J Bone Joint Surg Br 2007;89: 1218–24.
57. Gür E, Atesalp S, Basbozkurt M, et al. Treatment of complex calcaneal fractures with bony defects from land mine blast injuries with a circular external fixator. Foot Ankle Int 1999;20:37–41.
58. Tscherne H, Gotzen L. Pathophysiology and classification of soft tissue injuries associated with fractures. In: Tscherne H, Gotzen L, editors. Fractures with soft tissue injuries. Berlin: Spinger-Verlag; 1984. p. 1–9.
59. Hawkins LG. Fractures of the neck of the talus. J Bone Joint Surg Am 1970;52: 991–1002.
60. Canale ST, Kelly FB. Fractures of the neck of the talus. Long-term evaluation of seventy-one cases. J Bone Joint Surg Am 1978;60:143–56.
61. Vallier HA, Nork SE, Barei DP, et al. Talar neck fractures: results and outcomes. J Bone Joint Surg Am 2004;86-A:1616–24.
62. Young AF, Gwilym S, Cooke P, et al. Sub-optimal location of locking screw positioning in tibio-talo-calcaneal arthrodesis with an intramedullary device. Foot Ankle Surg 2007;13:122–5.
63. Santangelo JR, Glisson RR, Garras DN, et al. Tibiotalocalcaneal arthrodesis: a biomechanical comparision of multiplanar external fixation with intramedullary fixation. Foot Ankle Int 2008;29:936–41.
64. Hanson TW, Cracchiolo A. The use of a 95 degree blade plate and a posterior approach to achieve tibiotalocalcaneal arthrodesis. Foot Ankle Int 2002;23: 704–10.
65. Chodos MD, Parks BG, Schon LC, et al. Blade plate compared with locking plate for tibiotalocalcaneal arthrodesis: a cadaver study. Foot Ankle Int 2008;29: 219–24.
66. Myerson MS, Fisher RT, Burgess AR, et al. Fracture dislocations of the tarsometatarsal joints: end results correlated with pathology and treatment. Foot Ankle 1986;6:225–42.
67. Chiodo CP, Myerson MS. Developments and advances in the diagnosis and treatment of injuries to the tarsometatarsal joint. Orthop Clin North Am 2001;32:11–20.

Index

Note: Page numbers of article titles are in **boldface** type.

Foot Ankle Clin N Am 14 (2009) 589–616
doi:10.1016/S1083-7515(09)00070-9
1083-7515/09/$ – see front matter © 2009 Elsevier Inc. All rights reserved.

foot.theclinics.com

Moving?

Make sure your subscription moves with you!

To notify us of your new address, find your **Clinics Account Number** (located on your mailing label above your name), and contact customer service at:

Email: journalscustomerservice-usa@elsevier.com

800-654-2452 (subscribers in the U.S. & Canada)
314-447-8871 (subscribers outside of the U.S. & Canada)

Fax number: 314-447-8029

Elsevier Health Sciences Division
Subscription Customer Service
3251 Riverport Lane
Maryland Heights, MO 63043

Printed and bound by CPI Group (UK) Ltd, Croydon, CR0 4YY

03/10/2024

01040462-0007